M000113909

HUNGRY
for
SOLUTIONS

HUNGRY
for
SOLUTIONS

A MOTHER'S QUEST
TO DEFEAT HYPOTHALAMIC
AND CHILDHOOD OBESITY

MARCI SEROTA, RDN

Foreword by Thomas Inge, MD, PhD

BROWN BOOKS
PUBLISHING GROUP

Hungry for Solutions
A Mother's Quest to Defeat Hypothalamic and Childhood Obesity

Brown Books Publishing Group
16250 Knoll Trail Drive, Suite 205
Dallas, Texas 75248
www.BrownBooks.com
(972) 381-0009

A New Era in Publishing®

Publisher's Cataloging-In-Publication Data

Names: Serota, Marci.
Title: Hungry for solutions : a mother's quest to defeat hypothalamic and
    childhood obesity / Marci Serota, RDN.
Description: Dallas, Texas : Brown Books Publishing Group, [2018] | Includes
    bibliographical references.
Identifiers: ISBN 9781612542515
Subjects: LCSH: Obesity in children. | Hypothalamus--Diseases--
    Complications. | Serota, Marci--Family. | Mother and child.
Classification: LCC RJ399.C6 S47 2018 | DDC 618.92/398--dc23

ISBN 978-1-61254-251-5
LCCN 2018940001

Printed in the United States
10 9 8 7 6 5 4 3 2 1

For more information or to contact the author,
please go to www.CranioNutrition.com.

This book is dedicated to my children. Thank you for loving me unconditionally as I navigate my way through the perplexity of motherhood. You are both my pride and joy. JR, I won't always be here to guide you, but you will always have this book. Never forget: if you can do this, you can do anything. TJ, thank you for sharing me and making it possible for me to help so many people. This book is also dedicated to my Craniopharyngioma Facebook community. From me to you all, with love and hope.

Contents

Disclaimer

The nutritional information in this book is largely based on what has worked for my child, as well as my experience as a registered dietitian nutritionist. This book is meant to be used as a **general guideline for children (1) who have been diagnosed with hypothalamic obesity as a result of a brain tumor** *or other injury to the hypothalamus and* **(2)** who are morbidly obese. This food plan is *not* suitable or safe for children who have been diagnosed with kidney disease or liver failure with hepatic encephalopathy and/or who are or may be pregnant. **I am not a physician. Any and all recommendations, guidance, comments, and/or advice that I make regarding medications and/or dosage adjustments are solely recommendations for your child's physician to consider.**

Every child is different, and the carbohydrates, proteins, and calories that are provided in the food plans contained in this book are *not* appropriate or healthy for every child. **I do not advise implementing any new food plan without first obtaining permission and/or medical recommendation to implement such a food plan from your child's physician.** If your child is losing more than one to two pounds per week, then your child should increase their carbohydrate intake. Be aware that by following any food plan contained in this book, your child may develop certain micronutrient deficiencies (including but not limited to calcium, vitamin D, and/or certain B vitamins), and proper vitamin and mineral supplementation is recommended. In this regard, again, it is vital to consult your child's physician for explicit recommendations regarding proper supplementation of vitamins, minerals, and/or other. If your child is taking insulin, oral hypoglycemic agents, or other medication for diabetes mellitus, then your child's dosage may need to be adjusted by your child's physician to avoid low blood sugar. If your child is taking desmopressin for diabetes insipidus, your child's dosage will likely need to be decreased as your child loses weight to avoid/prevent low sodium levels. Again, it is imperative that you consult your child's physician for explicit recommendations for adjusting any such dosages of insulin, oral hypoglycemic agents, and/or desmopressin.

Foreword

Thomas Inge, MD, PhD

Hypothalamic obesity is a rare cause of severe obesity in children and adults. This form of obesity is a complex condition with a strong biological and biochemical basis. Unlike all other forms of obesity, this rare case is unique because it results from injury to critical areas of the deep brain (the hypothalamus) which control basic bodily functions such as weight regulation. The growth site of a rare brain tumor called a craniopharyngioma is so close to the hypothalamus that the tumor and/or the surgery necessary to remove it often damage the critical nerves and nerve pathways in the area, which results in a loss of the brain's ability to control appetite and weight gain.

The hypothalamus sends signals to the gut and other parts of the body and then receives feedback concerning satiety and energy stores from the gut and from fat cells. These signals travel back and forth, alerting the brain to hunger, fullness, any risk of starvation, or the need to continue or stop eating. For patients suffering damage to the hypothalamus, communication between the brain, the gut, and the fat stores have a critical missing component that is essential for central integration and relay—leaving the patient unable to regulate body weight.

As the hypothalamus is no longer participating in this delicate and critical communication, the patient will continue to eat insatiably (a condition called hyperphagia) with very little ability to consciously override the urge. The patient stores excess food as fat and seems never to feel full. In addition, damage to the hypothalamus may result in excess stimulation of insulin production. Not only will excess insulin increase appetite further, it also causes irritability and weight gain regardless of dietary restriction and exercise. This vicious cycle repeats daily as the patient gains more and more weight. Those suffering from hypothalamic obesity constantly feel that they are starving and can gain upwards of one or two pounds per week, even when attempting to maintain calorie-restricted diets and exercise routines.

The typical locations for safe fat storage (for instance, beneath the skin) are eventually overwhelmed, causing the body to store it in alternative places (in the muscles, liver, and around other important organs in the belly), which is often harmful to health. With this excess fat tucked into all of these important organs, the function of organs is impaired at the cellular level, and the result is poor health, including the development of fatty liver disease, type 2 diabetes, high blood pressure, high cholesterol, high triglycerides, heart disease, sleep apnea, and a poor quality of life.

Marci Serota's three-year-old son was diagnosed with a craniopharngioma in 2010 and, unfortunately, developed hypothalamic obesity. Despite Marci's training as a registered dietitian and her husband's medical degree, JR had grown severely obese by the time he was nine years old. With JR's health suffering and his liver enzymes multiplying dangerously, his gastroenterologist recommended that Marci and Dave look outside of their hometown for a pediatric surgeon experienced in treating hypothalamic obesity who might perform weight loss surgery.

The Serotas called me in January, 2016, to discuss their concerns about JR and their intent to explore a surgical treatment option for him. However, Marci also explained her desire to make one more full-court press with a special nutritional intervention before our scheduled clinic visit. I received a note from Marci in May of 2016 explaining the dietary and exercise program that she had created and implemented for JR. I was pleased to learn that JR's weight gain had been halted, and that, in fact, he had lost a significant amount of weight. Given that his health was also improving, we decided to cancel JR's appointment to allow Marci to continue treating him with her nutritional plan and lifestyle changes—the very plans that are outlined in this book. Two years later, I heard back from Marci that JR had lost forty pounds, that he was no longer severely obese, and that all of his blood tests had normalized. Significant weight loss in an obese child via diet and exercise is difficult and rare. Significant weight loss (without surgical intervention) in a child with hypothalamic obesity is almost unprecedented.

Marci and JR have accomplished something rarely seen without surgery. Marci's book details an effective, healthy, and satisfying approach to managing the daily food struggle for a child with hypothalamic obesity that is designed to dial down the intensity of hunger and improve health and quality of life. Marci's sensible approach to hypothalamic obesity is also applicable to other obese children, as it thoroughly addresses the root causes of not only this special form of obesity but childhood obesity in general.

While surgery may still be necessary for some children with hypothalamic obesity, it is only recommended in cases in which health is adversely affected and all other weight-loss measures have failed. The program that Marci details in *Hungry for Solutions* will help a great many families with children who suffer from hypothalamic obesity and may delay or prevent the need for bariatric surgery. *Hungry for Solutions* is an excellent source of guidance and inspiration for the parents of children struggling with obesity.

Thomas Inge, MD, PhD, FACS, FAAP
Professor of Surgery and Pediatrics,
University of Colorado, Denver
Chief of Pediatric Surgery and Director of Adolescent Bariatric Surgery,
Children's Hospital of Colorado, Aurora, Colorado

Preface

Let me begin by letting you know the most important thing—my child is happy. He is eleven years old now. He goes to school, he has good friends, and he loves art, music, science, swimming, Beyblade, and Pokémon. Yes, he developed hypothalamic obesity when he was only three years old. Yes, he has hyperphagia, and yes, at one point he was morbidly obese.

Let me explain where I was at when we got this diagnosis. I am a registered dietitian nutritionist and an avid and long-time yoga practitioner. Physical fitness and health have always been important to me. So when I was told that not only did my three-year-old son have a brain tumor but that this tumor would likely cause him to become obsessed with food and morbidly obese before he turned ten, it was a tough pill to swallow. Watching my child gain weight at a rapid pace was devastating. I worried about his health and all of the medical complications that I knew he would one day develop; I worried how it would affect him socially. I worried about being judged. Mostly, I worried that he would die at a very young age. He was well on his way. Fast forward eight years. JR has lost and kept off over forty pounds. His body mass index (BMI), which reached 36.5 before he was ten years old, is now down to 25. He has completely reversed the fatty liver disease that could have killed him. He is much more in control than I ever thought he'd be around food. His food cravings have decreased dramatically, and he has not regained any weight in the two years since starting his weight-loss journey, despite having grown over six inches. We did not accomplish this through surgery or fad diets. We did this with belief that it was possible; drive; solid, healthy nutritional know-how; and exercise. JR now has the knowledge and tools necessary to stay healthy for the rest of his life, in spite of his condition. He understands which foods trigger his hyperphagia and which foods are safe and in what amounts. My son is empowered and healthy now.

Author's Note

In 2010, when he was only three years old, JR was diagnosed with a rare type of brain tumor called a craniopharyngioma. Up to 55 percent of people treated for craniopharyngiomas develop a devastating condition called hypothalamic obesity with hyperphagia, which is characterized by high-fasting insulin levels, severely slowed metabolism, obsessive food-seeking behavior, rapid and unrelenting weight gain, and constant and overwhelming feelings of hunger. My son developed this condition near the age of four and subsequently gained over 140 pounds in a six-year period. I was unable to stop the rapid weight gain using traditional calorie- and portion-control methods. Although I tried constantly to control how much he was eating, he was much too young to understand and was constantly hungry, angry, combative, and unwilling to cooperate. We fought about food all the time, and he snuck extra food whenever he had the chance. I felt powerless and watched in horror for years as his health declined.

Everything that I read about hypothalamic obesity in the medical literature said that it is "unresponsive to diet and exercise." After a while, I started to believe that, and eventually I gave up fighting. The constant food policing and arguing about each morsel of food drained so much of my time and energy that I literally had nothing left for myself or the rest of my family. Around the time JR was eight years old, I decided that instead of fighting an uphill battle I wasn't winning anyway, I should try to shift my focus to creating happy memories for my children and our entire family rather than focusing exclusively on controlling JR's weight. I spent less time food policing and more time focusing on my younger child, who badly needed my attention. Although we were all happier for a while, JR's weight soon became dangerously high.

By age nine, JR weighed almost 180 pounds. He had high blood pressure, high cholesterol, and high triglycerides, and his liver had become clogged with fat. He was tired all of the time and fell asleep at school anytime he sat down. Even walking became painful and difficult. Finally, one of his specialists confirmed my worst fear: my son was headed down the path to liver failure. He understood that weight loss in a child with hypothalamic obesity is extremely challenging and recommended that we find a surgeon at a major pediatric obesity center who might agree to perform gastric bypass surgery to help him lose weight. We were terrified. My husband and I decided that it was time to shift all of our efforts back to controlling JR's weight and that we would do whatever it took to avoid bariatric surgery on our nine-year-old son. I quickly snapped out of my depressed, victim-mentality stupor and got to work.

Earlier in my career, I was fortunate enough to have spent three years mentoring with H. Theresa Wright, RD, MS, a cutting-edge dietitian in the Philadelphia area who has created a niche in food addiction. I suspected that a similar approach, with some tweaking specifically for HO, could work for hypothalamic obesity with hyperphagia.

I began to refamiliarize myself with nutrition intervention for conditions frequently seen in patients with HO, such as metabolic syndrome and type 2 diabetes. I finally decided to combine and modify the nutritional approaches used for food addiction, diabetes, and metabolic syndrome to create a plan that I hoped would at least stop JR's weight gain and maybe even result in some weight loss. I needed the whole family on board; I knew this would only work if we all did this as a team. My husband assured me that he was on board and would not bring any more food into the house without my approval. We also decided to hire a personal trainer to work out with JR to help him build some muscle and increase his slow metabolism as much as possible. I schooled my parents, who live nearby, as well as JR's teachers on his new plan.

I put the plan into place immediately, and within just five months, the improvement in JR's health was dramatic. He completely reversed his fatty liver disease and improved his lipid profile, decreasing his triglycerides by over two hundred points, lowering his LDL ("bad cholesterol") over fifty points, and raising his "good cholesterol" by thirteen points. The acanthosis nigricans (black spots on the body that signify hyperinsulinemia) disappeared. His blood pressure returned to normal. He began to have more energy. Once JR got used to the plan, we even stopped fighting about food so much, which was completely unexpected given his previously obsessive food-seeking behavior. The need to food police decreased significantly. He became self-motivated to exercise and stuck to his food plan.

The feeling of dread I had carried constantly for over six years was suddenly replaced by feelings of optimism and hope. It felt like a dream come true.

My intention for this book is that it will give people with hypothalamic obesity not only hope but also clear nutritional guidance for this devastating condition. I want to impress upon you that what I am recommending is not a "diet." It is a *lifestyle change* that will need to be continued indefinitely if you want to maintain what it can achieve—whether that is weight loss, an improved lipid profile, weight maintenance, or the reversal of fatty liver disease, type 2 diabetes, high blood pressure, metabolic syndrome, or sleep apnea. *Many* of the recommendations in this book can also be used as a solid guide for anyone struggling to find a permanent, effective, and safe way to achieve weight loss in any overweight child. Although I will be referring to hypothalamic obesity in children most of the time, know that if this plan can work for such an aggressive type of obesity, it can work even better for any obese child or adult who is struggling with their weight and cravings. This book is also intended to be a resource for nutrition professionals and physicians, giving them the tools they need to help their HO patients. I also wish to challenge and change the currently held medical opinion that hypothalamic obesity is "unresponsive to diet and exercise" and replace that with some solid nutritional advice and a more optimistic attitude for health-care professionals to transmit to their craniopharyngioma patients.

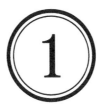

Introduction to Hypothalamic Obesity

What Are Hypothalamic Obesity (HO) and Hyperphagia?

Hypothalamic obesity is caused by damage to a part of the brain called the hypothalamus. The hypothalamus has many important jobs, including controlling metabolism, wake-sleep cycles (circadian rhythm), and the autonomic nervous system. Damage to the hypothalamus can result from either a brain tumor or from the surgery or radiation used to eradicate the brain tumor.

Damage to the hypothalamus causes the following problems, which lead to rapid weight gain and obesity that is stubborn to weight loss:

1. Disturbance of circadian rhythm, resulting in insomnia, hypersomnia, and secondary narcolepsy, causing excessive daytime sleepiness and lack of energy. Many individuals with hypothalamic damage are simply exhausted all of the time and therefore have a very hard time summoning the energy to exercise. They also tend to move around less, which results in fewer calories burned and decreased metabolism.

2. High-fasting insulin levels. Insulin is a hormone that is normally released into the bloodstream in response to eating carbohydrates. In a person with hypothalamic damage, their insulin levels are high even before they eat. Chronically high insulin levels cause weight gain, which results in insulin resistance, which makes weight loss that much more difficult.

3. Slow metabolism. Studies have shown that people with hypothalamic obesity burn significantly less energy while at rest than do obese people who do not have hypothalamic obesity. Even when calories are severely restricted, people with hypothalamic obesity often continue to gain weight.

4. Appetite regulation disturbances. People with hypothalamic damage do not receive a signal to their brains telling them that they feel "full." Therefore, they are always hungry, which often results in obsessive food-seeking behavior known as "hyperphagia." Children with HO with hyperphagia have been known to eat out of the trash, steal food from friends or stores, and even eat off the unattended plates of strangers.

In addition to causing hypothalamic damage, craniopharyngiomas often invade and destroy the pituitary gland, the "master gland." When one loses pituitary function, one's body stops making many important hormones, such as cortisol and thyroxine. Excessive cortisol replacement can further contribute to weight gain and prevent weight loss. Lack of pituitary function also causes secondary hypothyroidism, so metabolism takes another hit if thyroid replacement is not aggressive enough. As you can see, it is not surprising that people with hypothalamic damage gain a tremendous amount of weight very quickly and that this type of obesity is considered by the medical community to be "largely unresponsive to diet and exercise." It is not just a matter of simply overeating and underexercising. These patients have been reprogrammed to pump out insulin even in a fasting state and to store fat instead of burning it. Their brains do not get feedback that they have had enough to eat; they don't sleep well and are therefore too tired to exercise. If they have hyperphagia, they obsessively seek out, sneak, and steal food. The need to replace many of their hormones further insults a metabolism that is already in the gutter.

There is currently no generally accepted treatment for hypothalamic obesity. That means that there is no medication or surgery at this time that can cure this condition.

Diagnosis

Craniopharyngiomas are actually present at birth; they form in utero, tend to be very slow growing, and often go undiagnosed until they become so large that they have already damaged the hypothalamus. The signs and symptoms can range from behavioral problems to vision problems, weight loss or gain, slowed growth, and other endocrine problems, which are all often overlooked or attributed to other causes. Unfortunately, pediatricians and family practice physicians have not been trained to pick up on the early signs and symptoms of this rare type of brain tumor, and therefore, diagnosis often does not occur until these tumors have grown large enough to do irreparable damage to the eyes, brain, and body.

JR was late in meeting many of his developmental milestones (babbling, gesturing, sitting, crawling, walking, talking, etc.), so early on, I suspected that something was wrong. He was also extremely uncoordinated; he fell and tripped over things constantly. We took him to see a developmental pediatrician when he was fifteen months old, and he was diagnosed with a developmental coordination disorder and delayed speech. The doctor recommended that we start speech and occupational therapy and follow up with her in six months.

JR quickly caught up on his speech and language; however, he continued to have fine and gross motor difficulties. He also became increasingly anxious for no obvious reason, falling apart over small things like getting dressed in the morning, going to birthday parties, and having his hair washed. This was around the time that his brother was born, and I thought he was just having a hard time because of the new baby. I discussed his anxiety with his pediatrician, who suggested play therapy. Anxiety ran in our family, so I just assumed he came by it honestly, and maybe he did. I also thought that it was somehow my fault—that perhaps my exhaustion from caring for a newborn who didn't sleep had left me anxious and irritable. I set an intention to be more "in the moment," more patient, and less anxious about what could be wrong with him, and he began to relax a little bit, for a while.

Then seemingly unrelated issues began to pop up. I once noticed that half his smile did not match the other side, but then it went back to normal. Once, I was having a photo taken of him when suddenly, for a minute or two, he spaced out and stopped following directions, seeming confused. But then, just as suddenly, he went back to normal. He started crying each time we got in the car, complaining that the sunlight was too bright and hurt his eyes. I bought him sunglasses, thinking it was part of his sensory issues. I feared that all of these things were red flags for autism. It never entered my mind that he could have a brain tumor. With the exception of the photosensitivity, there is no way to know if any of these other symptoms I have mentioned thus far were, in fact, related to his tumor.

When JR was three, I noticed that he was suddenly shorter than peers he had previously towered over and that his scapula bones were sticking out. He had also fallen from the 90th percentile to the 65th percentile in height on his growth chart. I asked the doctor about this at his check-up; I was told that sometimes children move around on their growth curve. As JR neared his fourth birthday, even the light indoors became too much for him, and he wanted to wear sunglasses inside too. Then the headaches started. JR would come into our room in the middle of the night crying that his head hurt, but then he'd wake up feeling fine the next day. His play therapist felt that these nighttime-only headaches were just anxiety and instructed us to send him back to his room. She said that letting him come to bed with us would just worsen his anxiety. I was up multiple times a night with JR and his little brother, who still wasn't sleeping through the night. I desperately needed sleep, so I listened to her. I will never get over the guilt I still feel for sending JR back to bed, night after night, crying with a headache, to be alone in his room with what was actually hydrocephalus—increased pressure from fluid accumulating in his brain from a brain tumor.

Next, JR's preschool teacher called to tell me that JR had crawled into her lap and fallen asleep during recess that day, which was very odd. A few days later, he vomited; we thought he must have a virus, and so we kept him home for the next few days. *There was no fever.* The doctor agreed that it was likely just a virus and told us to bring him back if he wasn't feeling better in a few days. JR seemed to get better for a few days. He went back to school, played baseball when he got home, and even went to a birthday party. Then the headaches returned, and he suddenly started napping after school. Again, this was odd; JR hadn't taken an afternoon nap since he was two years old. Then he started taking two naps a day. Finally, my husband, Dave, who is a physician, confided in me that he was worried that JR might have a brain tumor. It was a Saturday evening, so I immediately called the on-call nurse, who told me that it was probably a virus and to tell my husband to "look for horses, not zebras." The next day, we had a birthday party at our house for my youngest son's first birthday; JR slept through the entire thing. He vomited again the next morning, so we took him back to the pediatrician. He still had no fever, and his white blood cell count was normal, so his doctor ordered a CT scan of his brain.

Dave went into the scan with our son while I sat in the waiting room with my mother. He actually saw the brain tumor on the screen, confirming his worst fears. I knew the second they came out of that scan, before he said a word; I could see it written all over his face. I somehow maintained my composure, asked my mother to take JR home, and told her that we'd be there shortly. Dave and I stepped out into the lobby just outside of the imaging center and watched JR get into my mom's car and drive away. I was stunned. Numb. I stood there, knowing my three-year-old baby had a brain tumor but unable to allow the information to penetrate my soul—unable to do anything except hold my husband and tremble uncontrollably as he sobbed, our world crashing down around us.

Treatment Options

We had very little time to grieve. That came later. Years later. My husband and my father, also a physician, took JR's scan straight to a radiologist, got a diagnosis of hydrocephalus and craniopharyngioma, and arranged a meeting with a pediatric neurosurgeon before our pediatrician had even gotten the results of the scan. We had about one hour between the time we arrived home from the CT scan and the time we had to leave to meet with the neurosurgeon and discuss our options. I finally broke down and cried as quietly as I could in the bathroom so that JR wouldn't hear me. We told him very little. Just that we needed to pack his suitcase and special blanket, go see a doctor about his headaches, and maybe stay at the hospital for a little while until he felt better. That was the last time I cried about it for almost two years.

The neurosurgeon explained to us that, although the tumor itself was benign and could certainly be removed, it was essentially "a good tumor that was growing in a very bad location." It was located on JR's hypothalamus, had invaded his pituitary gland, and was pressing on his optic nerve, which was the reason for the photosensitivity. Craniopharyngiomas can be solid- or mixed-type tumors that sprout fluid-filled cysts. It was the cystic component that was causing the headaches, vomiting, heightened anxiety, and lethargy. The doctor expressed concern that removing the solid portion of the tumor could damage JR's hypothalamus and cause morbid obesity and obsessive food-seeking behavior. Suddenly, JR's craniopharyngioma didn't seem so benign anymore.

Our surgeon's plan was to leave the solid portion of the tumor alone for now, to place a reservoir under the scalp—which would allow him to drain the fluid-filled cyst—and to later place a radioactive isotope into the cyst to collapse the cystic portion of the tumor. JR needed to have that fluid drained emergently, so we went ahead with that surgery. This gave us some time to think and do some research before making any bigger treatment decisions.

Dave and I were just not comfortable with the next phase of the plan. We worried that a radioactive isotope could leak out of the cyst and into JR's brain, causing more problems. Plus, we learned that craniopharyngiomas often sprout multiple cysts . . . What then? More surgery, more drains, and more radioactive isotopes? We didn't want to go against our neurosurgeon's advice—he had a fabulous reputation and had already operated on JR, and we were incredibly grateful to him. However, we were concerned that leaving a tumor in his brain that not only would continue to grow but was already wrapped around JR's optic nerve could cause him to go blind. Plus, there was a chance that the tumor itself, if left to grow, would eventually cause hypothalamic obesity anyway.

We asked for a second meeting with the neurosurgeon, explaining our fears. We wanted to know what he intended to do with the solid portion of the tumor after the radioactive isotope had collapsed the cyst. Surgery to remove the tumor? Radiation? Both? He was not specific about his plan for treating the solid portion of the tumor. Again, we pressed him for his exact plan, and he finally gave us a vague response of "possibly radiation, maybe resection," leaving us with even more questions and even more uncomfortable. If he was planning to maybe remove the tumor anyway, why wait? He arranged for us to meet with radiation oncology to find out more about the possibility of radiation. The radiation oncologist told us that craniopharyngiomas are very resistant to radiation. Therefore, twenty-five rounds of gamma knife radiation to JR's brain would be necessary to stop the tumor from growing any larger, each session being one and a half hours long and each under general anesthesia. Dave and I both agreed that repeated radiation to our three-year-old's brain scared us more than surgery and the possibility of hypothalamic obesity. We knew that radiation could cause secondary tumors and negatively affect JR's cognition. Our

neurosurgeon suggested that we get a second opinion to explore resection (removing the tumor surgically) if we were unsure.

Dave called pediatric neurosurgeons all over the country to explore
our options. They all disagreed with one another. There was much
disagreement among pediatric neurosurgeons about how to treat
craniopharyngiomas in a way that prevented or delayed the onset of
hypothalamic obesity and preserved quality of life for the patient. One
camp felt that completely removing the tumor was the way to go. The
other camp felt that treating the cysts as they arose and then doing
radiation and/or partial resection would provide a better quality of life,
at least for a while longer. Both treatment options carried risks of serious
complications and side effects.

We read as many studies as we could find on treating craniopharyngiomas and on hypothalamic obesity. We found a wonderful,
compassionate pediatric neurosurgeon who spent literally hours on
the phone with us, answering all of our questions, and who also had a
tremendous amount of experience resecting craniopharyngiomas with
a relatively low incidence of hypothalamic obesity. We understood
that by removing the tumor, there was a chance JR would end up with
hypothalamic obesity and hyperphagia, but we felt that JR's chances of
developing severe hypothalamic obesity would be much lower going
with a surgeon with a lot of experience resecting this type of tumor. We
felt strongly that curing the tumor—versus repeated and painful drain-
ing of the cyst, more surgeries to place more drains, and twenty-five
rounds of radiation to our three-year-old's developing brain—was our
best option, even with the increased risk of HO from the surgery.

We discussed our options ad nauseam with our new neurosurgeon, our
pediatrician, our extended family, and each other and then made the most
monumental, agonizing decision of our lives—to have the tumor removed.
We got on a plane and headed out of town, praying that JR would be both
cured and spared the dreaded hypothalamic obesity and hyperphagia.

Despite the difficulty of the next six years, we have never questioned
our treatment choice. After almost eight years, there has been no sign
of tumor recurrence, and no further treatment has been necessary thus

far. Craniopharyngiomas are notorious for regrowing, so the fact that it hasn't come back is a credit to the skill and competency of JR's wonderful neurosurgeon. Although JR did end up developing hypothalamic obesity and hyperphagia, it is thankfully far from severe, and we have figured out how to manage it and keep JR's weight and appetite under control. We continue to be grateful that JR has not required additional brain surgeries and treatment thus far. Although JR has to have MRIs of his brain to check for tumor recurrence on a yearly basis, the likelihood of recurrence decreases substantially after the first few years of being tumor-free.

Surgery

It was gut wrenching to have to kiss my son goodbye and watch as he was rolled away to surgery, knowing full well that a different child might come out when it was over. The surgery took eight hours. The job of going through the brain to reach the area where the tumor was located and then removing the tumor without damaging the surrounding optic nerve, blood vessels, and hypothalamus had to be painstakingly meticulous. Recovery from brain surgery is difficult, and in a three-year-old, it's even harder. Once the surgery was over, the stress finally overwhelmed me. I had been so strong and had not cried, had not doubted, had not let myself entertain any fears that JR might die or that we'd made the wrong choice. Shortly after the doctor came out of the OR to tell us that the surgery was over and he thought he'd gotten all of the tumor out, my body finally gave out; I became so ill that I had to go to the ER twice while JR was recovering in the intensive care unit. They told me it was probably food poisoning, but I knew it was stress. I was sick for weeks. I couldn't eat. I went down three dress sizes in the month that JR was in the hospital. But there was no time for me to rest and recover; although I had plenty of family there to be with JR, I was the one he wanted. JR was terrified of all the sights and sounds and constant taking of vitals and poking and prodding from caregivers, especially the IV he had to have in his arm.

After a month in the hospital, we finally brought JR home and began the rehabilitation process. He had been in bed for almost a month and was very weak, depressed, and scared; even climbing the stairs to his room was too much for him. He had been on several courses of high-dose steroids, and he looked and felt like a different person. All of this caused him a tremendous amount of anxiety. We were told to expect short-term memory loss, which meant JR couldn't remember that he'd just eaten. Plus, he was ravenous from the high-dose steroids he had received in the hospital, so this caused further distress. For weeks, all he did was sleep, eat, and cry.

Losing Control: Living with Hyperphagia

JR began to gain weight very quickly, but we hoped and prayed that it was the high-dose steroids from the surgery and not hypothalamic obesity. Within a few weeks, JR began to ask for food constantly. He could not seem to go more than twenty minutes without asking for something to eat. When we told him that it wasn't time to eat yet, he would get angry and cry.

After a year or so of this, when JR was five, we eventually had to accept the fact that something in his brain had changed. Prior to the craniopharyngioma, we were able to keep foods such as low-sugar dry cereal, crackers, pretzels, frozen waffles, and the occasional treat in the house, and overeating was never an issue. Now these foods became an overwhelming temptation to JR, and while his portion sizes began to grow, the complaints of hunger never ceased. I stopped bringing these foods into the house for a long time. It didn't seem to matter; he would eat enormous amounts of "healthy food" each day and began sneaking food to his room. When I say "enormous amounts of food," I mean an entire loaf of sliced whole-wheat bread or five to six apples at a time. He would slyly polish off the remains of any unattended plate. Admittedly, desserts and sweets sometimes made their way into the house when we entertained company and after Halloween or other holidays. We tried to keep them out of his reach, but I'd always find crumbs and wrappers in his room. He would sneak down to the kitchen in the middle of the night, and every morning, I was devastated to find that he'd consumed large amounts of food while we slept. We tried to lock the fridge at night to prevent this, but our fridge had french doors with the freezer on the bottom, and we were not able to lock the freezer securely enough; JR was able to squeeze his arm in there and get to frozen waffles and raw hot dogs. We finally had to buy a refrigerator with side-by-side doors.

Any attempt I made to redirect him or limit his portion sizes and access to food ended in tantrums. My entire life became about food policing and trying to keep JR from overeating. It was a full-time job. The second I left the kitchen to use the facilities or to attend to my younger son, JR would sneak food from the kitchen, take it up to his room, and hide it for later. Birthday parties and social gatherings became a nightmare with the cake and juice and candy favors. He was so young, he just didn't understand why he was not allowed to eat all of the same foods as the other children and why some were permitted juice, second helpings of cake, and candy as they walked out the door when he was only permitted one small piece of cake with water and no candy. He'd throw a tantrum in front of all of the children and their parents, making a scene, and then shove forbidden food into his mouth before I could get it out of his hands. I would react angrily, and we'd have to leave parties abruptly, both of us crying. Restaurants were impossible because of the enormous portion sizes of calorie-laden food. He wanted to eat all of the food on the plate, no matter how big, and he argued and cried and kicked when we told him that he could only eat half and save the rest for another time. The only solution was to avoid social functions that involved food and restaurants, which left us isolated and alone. Family meals deteriorated into a war zone. At each and every meal, my younger son would sit quietly, picking at his food, while the haggling and arguing and crying took place, and when I couldn't take it any longer, I'd lose my temper and start yelling at JR.

We tried to keep him active. We enrolled him in a soccer class for exercise twice a week, plus physical and occupational therapy three times per week, which helped a little. But as he got older, he stopped wanting to play soccer. I was exhausted from the emotional and physical stress that had been going on for years. We still had a full schedule of endocrinologists, pediatricians, gastroenterologists, play therapy, occupational therapy, speech therapy, and driving back and forth to two different schools that were nowhere near my home. After a full day of school, JR was exhausted, and we could not get him to exercise. I had been living in "survival mode" for four years, and I had nothing left. I just did not have the energy to fight with him about exercise as well as food, so eventually he stopped getting exercise.

Rock Bottom

Before diagnosis, JR was three years old and weighed thirty-three pounds. By the time he was nine years old, he weighed almost 180 pounds and was morbidly obese and sick with fatty liver disease, sleep apnea, high blood pressure, and high triglyceride levels. To say that I was devastated would be an understatement.

It had been a living hell for five years of our lives. The brain tumor was scary, but at least there were treatment options and the hope that it wouldn't regrow. With the ensuing hypothalamic obesity, no one offered us any hope or knew how to help us. The hyperphagia felt like a prison sentence because there was no end in sight. JR had always been a strong-willed child and could argue and negotiate until my head started spinning. He attempted to negotiate portion sizes at every meal and every snack, every day, often wearing me down until I either lost my temper with him or just let him eat more than I was comfortable with. After I'd lose my temper, I'd be wracked with guilt because I knew that it wasn't his fault. No words can describe enduring your child whining and crying to you all day long, every day, that he is hungry and having him hate you for withholding food from him.

As he grew older, JR began to hate me with every fiber of his being, and our entire relationship deteriorated to the point that the only things we talked about with each other were what he could and could not eat and in what amounts. On top of that, I felt guilty for allowing my need to try to control JR's eating steal literally all of my attention away from his younger brother, TJ. Life felt so hard, so exhausting, and so miserable that I couldn't even look at food anymore; I completely lost my appetite and still have a hard time enjoying food to this day. All I wanted to do was sleep away as much of the day as possible. My life felt like *Groundhog Day*, and I deeply resented having to wake up every morning and repeat the same miserable experience day after day after day.

We were up against something powerful; JR's brain had been reprogramed to direct him to eat as much as possible and no longer received any feedback from his body telling him that he was full. His metabolism was deranged, his pancreas was pumping out too much insulin, and he fought us tooth and nail when we tried to restrict his intake of food. It is no wonder that we became so discouraged that we began to accept that we were powerless to defeat this condition. I really had tried for a good many years. In addition to the constant food policing, I measured his portion sizes on a food scale, we stopped going out to eat or to parties, and I tried not to keep junk in the kitchen. I even took JR to see two different pediatric dietitians over the years, conceding that I obviously didn't know what to do. They didn't know what to do either. I asked doctors to prescribe stimulant medications, hoping that might help. It didn't. No matter how hard I tried to get my son to make good choices, he just kept sneaking food and gaining weight.

All of the fighting, yelling, crying, guilt, and social isolation created an extremely toxic family environment. Food permeates every part of American life—all fun activities and venues, family gatherings, and even religious holidays revolve around food. Since we could no longer be a part of it, we stayed at home most of the time, and our home was not a pleasant place to be.

Eventually, and not surprisingly, my younger son developed serious food aversions. I put him into play therapy to work through his frustration with the situation and feeding therapy to help with the food aversions. Once it was clear that TJ was being negatively impacted by all of the dysfunction surrounding food, I decided that we could not go on like this any longer. I was spending all of my time and energy fighting an uphill battle that I was clearly losing, and we were all miserable. I decided that it was time to put TJ's needs—and my own—above my need to keep JR from gaining more weight. I again began to buy foods that TJ would eat: Goldfish, pretzels, and Kashi Heart to Heart cereal. I tried to keep JR from eating them but was rarely successful.

I decided to redefine my idea of what it meant to be a "good mother." Instead of "I am a good mother because I keep JR healthy," I tried to think, "I am a good mother because I create happy memories for both of my children." It was such a relief to let up on the food policing for a while and to be able to devote that time to TJ and to myself. I began to spend more time outside, taking the dog for long walks and visiting with neighbors, and gave more of my attention to TJ rather than standing guard in the kitchen all of the time. For a while, we were all happier, and life seemed bearable again. I tried to ignore the fact that JR was getting bigger and bigger and growing sicker and sicker, telling myself that if I could not change his destiny, I could at least make the time that we had together happier, even if that meant we would have less time. I still tried to guide him to make good choices, but I tried not to let it consume my life. I continued in this vein for a year and a half, until I received the results of one of JR's routine blood tests and noticed that his liver enzymes had doubled.

I knew that meant his liver was literally turning into fat and would eventually fail. I felt completely powerless to stop it. I made an appointment for JR to see a pediatric gastroenterologist, but I could not bring myself to show up for the appointment; I knew what the doctor would say, and I couldn't bear to hear it. So I asked Dave to go instead. He returned home from the appointment badly shaken. The doctor had suggested that we try to find a pediatric surgeon who would be willing to perform gastric bypass surgery on JR. Dave argued that there wasn't a surgeon in the country who would do such an operation on a nine-year-old child. "You don't know that," was the physician's response. This time, I wasn't numb—I was hysterical. A doctor only recommends bariatric surgery on a nine-year-old child when things have reached a critical point. The threat of losing JR was real now. My worst fears were becoming reality.

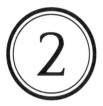

Hope and Intention

The Cost of Losing Hope

After it became clear that JR had hypothalamic obesity, I often complained to his many doctors about how difficult it was to stop the rapid weight gain, even for a mother who was a nutritionist. They were not able to offer me anything other than sympathy. Hypothalamic obesity is one of the most frustrating conditions for doctors to deal with, because there is no effective treatment. No medications can turn the constant hunger off. Doctors are simply at a loss for what to do to help these patients. I myself had received zero training on this condition. When I read over the medical literature on hypothalamic obesity and hyperphagia, I heard the same messages in article after article: "this type of obesity is unresponsive to diet and exercise" and "weight loss efforts are unsuccessful."

When all hope is lost, the natural consequence is to stop trying so hard and to stop looking for new solutions. Losing hope and accepting defeat basically cemented JR's future as a morbidly obese child who would need gastric bypass surgery by the age of nine or die at an early age.

Around first grade, the other kids began teasing JR about his weight. I remember him asking me, "Mommy, if I work very hard, do you think I can lose weight?"

I didn't know how to respond. I was afraid to get his hopes up; my own hope had already been shattered, and I had already resigned myself to the idea that there was nothing more we could do. After all, two other dietitians and I had failed to control his weight gain. I knew that if JR and I lived in a vacuum, I could have effected some weight loss—but we didn't live in a vacuum. We lived in the real world, with siblings and friends who seemed to eat whatever they wanted; where high-carb, high-sugar, processed food was ubiquitous and giant portion sizes inescapable; where teachers gave students candy for positive reinforcement; where schedules were full, time and energy for exercise was limited, and JR's drive to exercise was nonexistent; and where JR was a strong-willed, angry, chronically hungry young child. In that context, I had clearly failed.

So I did the most detrimental thing possible: I relayed my acceptance of the status quo to JR by responding, "I don't know. Maybe? Maybe not?" I didn't want to discourage him, but I could not bear to give him false hope either. He burst into tears, and I held him, crying too.

The Power of Hope and Intention

Soon after JR's gastroenterologist suggested we look into gastric bypass surgery, JR's psychologist told him, "JR, even though it may be difficult for you to control your thoughts about food, you do have *some* control over how much you choose to eat." I happened to be in the room with them during this particular session, and I was surprised to hear her say this. How could she say that to him without really knowing whether or not it was true? I loved what I was hearing and so wanted to believe it, but was she giving my son unrealistic expectations? Then I remembered something that I had once learned about from my Ayurveda practitioner—the power of setting an intention.

If you can visualize what you want actually happening, and if you never stop believing it is possible, then *it will happen*. If you believe that you can't, then you are doomed before you even start. That precious, brilliant psychologist changed our mind-set and JR's trajectory forever that day by giving us hope that JR did have some control over his hyperphagia. And guess what? He does! We had not seen any evidence of it up to that point; he had never before flexed his control "muscle." But it was there, latent, waiting to be activated. After we set our intention that we would defeat this HO monster that had taken over our lives, JR proved time and time again that he indeed had some control over his actions and choices with regard to food! Changing his habits and rewiring his usual response to food took practice and time, but it was absolutely possible—even for a child with HO and hyperphagia who had all of the cards stacked against him.

Intention starts with a goal—a visualization of what you want to achieve—along with the dogged determination to make it happen. Once we got most of the sugar and man-made food out of his system, JR began to demonstrate control over his impulses to eat everything in sight. I can't tell you how many times since we have begun this weight-loss journey that JR has found food left out by his brother, brought it to me, and said, "Mom, I am afraid I am going to eat this . . . Can you get rid of it?" He has also brought home food from school countless times (on days I let him order "hot lunch") and proudly showed me that he did not eat all of it because the portion size was too big. Of course, sometimes he chose to eat it all, but that began happening less and less often and is now actually quite infrequent. His belief that he can control his hyperphagia empowers him to resist overeating more and more often. Of course, this doesn't mean controlling his impulses to eat won't be a struggle for the rest of his life. But he will always know that he does have the power to say no to food and that he can access that willpower at any time. So please don't buy into the "there is nothing I can do, I am doomed" mentality. It doesn't have to be true for you! If you want it badly enough, and if you believe that it is possible, I am here to tell you that you *can* make it happen.

I am not trying to minimize anyone's struggles. There is a spectrum of hypothalamic obesity, and there is definitely a spectrum of response to diet and lifestyle change. Mild and moderate hypothalamic obesity will likely respond best to diet, exercise, and lifestyle change. There are those with severe HO who might not lose any weight, but that doesn't mean that they cannot improve their health and/or stop or slow their weight gain. That is not defeat! That can be the difference between developing diabetes or not, the difference between dying of a heart attack at a young age or not. There is always a win to be gained; there is always some power that you have over this—but only if you believe it is possible, work as hard as you can, and never give up. HO is not a black-and-white situation, so please don't accept defeat, not ever. Most importantly, teach your HO child that they do have *some* control over their hyperphagia, even if you don't really believe it. Make them believe it, and praise them every time they display the slightest hint of it. And please do not punish them or make them feel bad when they don't.

What I wish doctors would say to their patients with HO is this: "Controlling your weight will be hard, *but not necessarily impossible*. You will have to change your entire family's eating and lifestyle, but there is a chance you can control this if you work very hard and believe in yourself. However, if you accept defeat before you even try—if you are not willing to work very hard and do whatever it takes—the HO will win." A little hope can go a long way.

Taking Back Control

My first reaction to the news that JR needed gastric bypass surgery at nine years old was to hide under the covers and cry. Dave, once again, took a more pragmatic approach. He stated our intention: "We are going to do whatever it takes to help JR lose some weight so that he doesn't have to have this surgery." His determination was contagious and immediately made me feel empowered. I realized that I knew exactly how we would accomplish this. I had always known; I had just lacked hope, intention, and, most importantly, drive.

The first problem was that although we had tried to get JR to change the way he was eating, Dave, TJ, and I hadn't made any real effort to change the way we were eating. Stupidly, it had not occurred to us that expecting a young child to completely give up certain foods while the rest of us were eating them was not only unrealistic but downright counterproductive.

It was tricky, because JR's brother was a very picky eater, I struggled with my appetite, and Dave worked all day without eating anything and then sometimes stopped at the grocery store, ravenous, after work, bringing home foods that he thought were healthy but really weren't. So although we weren't eating Doritos and donuts, "healthier" processed foods like pretzels, organic tortilla chips, "whole-grain" Goldfish, and dry cereal did sometimes make their way into our home. We would try to hide them from JR and eat them when he wasn't around, but he always found them and ate them too. Let's be real—the other reason we bought these foods, other than the fact that we could not see the forest for the trees, was that we were just as attached to these processed foods as everyone else is. It doesn't matter that I am a nutritionist or that Dave is a doctor; we are humans first, and this was the way we had always eaten. Our unconscious attitude was that since we were able to eat these foods without obvious consequences (namely, we didn't gain any weight from doing so), why should we have to give them up just because JR did? He was the one with the weight problem, after all, not us. Clearly, we would have to make some major changes in our eating if we expected JR to do the same.

I told Dave, "We will have to get all of the processed food out of the house and eat only natural foods. You won't be able to bring food into the house that I don't approve. *We are all going to have to eat the same way that we make JR eat. We have to do this together, as a team, or it won't work.*" I suggested we hire a personal trainer to work out with JR. I knew it would be expensive, and we'd have to get him there several times a week, so I would need help with that.

"Fine," Dave replied. "Done." We were in business.

I began to communicate with other craniopharyngioma survivors via Facebook about what, if anything, worked for them. Time and time again, I heard the same message: "Cut the carbs, cut the carbs, cut the carbs." I hesitated to put JR on a very low-carb diet because, in my experience, people who follow such a plan lose a lot of weight quickly, but only the most self-disciplined are able to stick with a very low-carb diet for more than a year, and once they start eating more carbs, they gain back more weight than where they began. Also, I knew my child, and I needed his cooperation for this to work. I knew that if my plan were too restrictive, he wouldn't cooperate. I needed to come up with something slightly different.

Next I thought about the physiological factors that were contributing to his weight gain. Other than hyperphagia / food seeking / never feeling full, what was contributing to his weight that I could actually control? I knew that JR's body was putting out way too much insulin, not only because he was obese but primarily because of the metabolic derangements caused by the damage to his hypothalamus. I knew that he would not lose weight as long as his insulin levels continued to be high. So, I reasoned, if carbs triggered insulin secretion, then if I limited the amount of carbs he ate at any one time, I could potentially minimize his insulin production.

Since hyperphagia closely resembles food addiction, I wondered if the food-addiction model of removing the man-made, processed carbs might have the added benefit of calming the food cravings and obsessive food-seeking behaviors seen in patients with hyperphagia. I also refreshed my memory on nutritional intervention for metabolic syndrome, which JR was at high risk for developing. I decided that combining the nutritional interventions used for diabetes (carb counting), metabolic syndrome (strictly limiting sugar and carbs), and food addiction (removing flour, sugar, and man-made foods), with the addition of some elements specific to patients with hyperphagia, would be the best approach to take. I wrote out a food plan, got rid of all the processed food in my house, and made an appointment with a trainer who worked with young children. I explained to JR what we needed to do and why; he became hysterical and thought I planned to starve him. I explained that I needed him to trust me, that he would be eating frequently, and that I would not starve him. I added that if he lost twenty pounds, we'd take him to Disneyland. He stopped crying and actually became excited. Now we had a solid plan and, just as importantly, JR's cooperation. My plan not only worked but saved my son's life, avoided the need to have gastric bypass surgery, and improved his quality of life and that of our entire family.

Ingredients for Success

1. We avoid almost all "man-made" and high-temptation foods (sugar, bread, pasta, and all über-processed foods) and do not keep them in our home.

2. We limit JR's carbohydrate intake to roughly 12–20* grams of carb at each meal and snack to minimize JR's insulin secretion as much as possible. *I did not include his intake of nonstarchy vegetables in this number.*

3. Ninety-five percent of the carbohydrates that we eat are "nature-made carbs." In other words, the majority of our carbohydrate intake comes from carbs that we could grow ourselves if necessary. Most nature-made carbs are high in fiber, which slows digestion and insulin response.[1] See a list of nature-made carbs in the "Nature-Made Carb Choices" section later in the book. Bread and pasta are *not* nature-made carbs.

4. We limit fruit intake to 4 ounces maximum, no more than two to three times per day, to decrease triglyceride levels and sugar cravings. We avoid dried fruit except in *very* small quantities.

5. We eat as many nonstarchy vegetables as we like in between meals and snacks and sometimes add an extra ounce or two of protein or

---

1. L. Te Morenga, P. Docherty, S. Williams, and J. Mann, "The Effect of a Diet Moderately High in Protein and Fiber on Insulin Sensitivity Measured Using the Dynamic Insulin Sensitivity and Secretion Test (DISST)," *Nutrients* 9, no. 12 (2017): 1291, doi:10.3390/nu9121291.

healthy fat if there will be more than three hours between meals and snacks.

6. We do not eat anything that contains more than 5 grams of sugar per serving, unless it is intended to be a dessert. The less sugar, the better.

7. We weigh or measure everything JR eats, except for nonstarchy vegetables. This prevents portion sizes from slowly growing over time. Invest in a good food scale.

8. We do not eat out more than once a week, and we choose restaurants very carefully. We do not go to restaurants that are not geared toward healthy eating. We agree on an acceptable entrée before we even go to the restaurant so that there is no arguing or tears at dinner.

9. We have a personal trainer work out with JR twice a week, thirty minutes per session. In addition, JR swims or walks a few times a week. Exercise is a must.

10. We offer positive reinforcement for weight loss. It will be very difficult for a child to lose weight if they won't cooperate. You will need to set a weight-loss goal (a reasonable amount of weight to lose, like maybe five or even ten pounds) and offer positive reinforcement for achieving that goal—something they really want.

11. Notice I use the word "we" in most of the preceding tips. Our entire family eats the same way and exercises too (though not always together). I cannot stress how important it is that the entire family does this together. The portion sizes can be different for those who do not need to lose weight. The chances for success are infinitely greater if the entire family does this together. If not, then the child feels punished and will likely be resentful and resistant. Trust me:

whatever is off limits to the child who needs to lose weight must be off limits to everyone else, at least when the child is present.

12. I've been honest with JR. I let him know that his doctor said that he is going to get very sick and could even die if we don't make all of the above changes and stick to them for the rest of his life. Tough love.

Numbers 13 and 14 are only appropriate for children with a diagnosis of hypothalamic obesity and hyperphagia.

13. We addressed JR's low energy levels. First we put him on Adderall, a stimulant medication that was recommended by a pediatric obesity specialist, for a limited period of time. Stimulants are notorious for decreasing appetite. In our experience, however, Adderall did not dramatically decrease JR's appetite, but it seemed to help a little bit. Where we did see a big difference was in his energy levels. It gave him the energy he desperately needed to exercise, and that is very important. Note: once JR's weight loss plateaued, we discontinued the Adderall, due to unpleasant side effects, and instead started him on liothyronine (T3), another thyroid replacement hormone. He tolerates the liothyronine very well, and it seems to have an even better effect on his energy levels. Note that liothyronine is only appropriate for children with a diagnosis of secondary hypothyroidism. Please discuss with your doctor whether any medication to increase energy or decrease appetite is safe or appropriate for your HO child.

14. We locked the pantry and refrigerator twenty-four seven between meals and at night. Fortunately, locking access to food twenty-four seven is no longer necessary. We did this for about two years, and it wasn't easy. More on that later in the book.

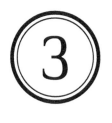

Background

Sugar

Sugar is the enemy. There are many types of sugar: sucrose, a.k.a. table sugar, which comes from sugarcane; fructose, a simple sugar found naturally in fruits, vegetables, and honey; and lactose, which is the sugar present in cow's milk. Although fructose and lactose do cause problems when eaten in excess and should be limited, especially in children with hypothalamic obesity, I am not referring to these types of sugar. When I use the word "sugar," I am mainly talking about processed sugars such as sucrose and high-fructose corn syrup.

Sugar is one of the worst things for any animal to consume, hypothalamic obesity or not. Sucrose increases food cravings and causes insulin spikes, which direct our bodies to store fat rather than burn it for energy, which causes more hunger and cravings for more sugar! Processed fructose and even fructose from fruit juice is converted directly to fat in the liver, raising triglycerides, causing inflammation and, if consumed regularly, fatty liver disease. High-fructose corn syrup is the absolute worst thing you can put into your body if you are trying to lose weight or avoid weight gain.

Sugar is also highly addictive. It alters our brain chemistry and makes us feel really good, much like recreational drugs do, triggering us to want to eat more and more and making many of us feel out of control. *Sugar is basically an easy-to-access "drug" that millions of children and adults use to manage their feelings all day long. Children become addicted to sugar at a very young age.*

Sugar is everywhere, hiding in almost everything we eat. Sugar has many different names: glucose, dextrose, cane juice crystals, agave, evaporated cane juice, malt, caramel color, high-fructose corn syrup, and ribose, just to name a few! Reading the ingredient list of any food you purchase is very important in limiting one's sugar intake. You will be surprised to find that the food companies have put sugar in your deli meats, bread, crackers, potato chips, french fries, chicken nuggets, cereal, condiments, pretzels, popcorn, hamburgers, hot dogs—*everything.* They do this to extend the shelf life of their products and so that their foods will taste so good, and make you feel so good, that you cannot stop eating their products, therefore ensuring that you will keep buying more of what they are selling. *High-sugar, über-processed food is like crack to children with hyperphagia.*

High Sugar, Über-Processed "Nonfoods"–How Did We Get Here?

Long ago, before the Industrial Revolution, humans ate and lived very differently than we do now. People grew their own food; raised their own hens; milked their own cows; plucked their own chickens; hunted, gutted, and cleaned their own game; grew and harvested their own wheat; ground their own flour; and baked their own bread. They burned calories all day long, washing their clothes by hand, sewing their own clothes, and walking to school. Children helped with house chores and in the fields after school and on the weekends, and people were able to utilize most of the calories that they ate. They also ate mostly whole, unprocessed, nature-made food. Sugar was expensive and reserved for a very special treat that few could afford.

Enter the Industrial Revolution, and, nutritionally speaking, things went downhill very fast. People moved to cities and began buying most of their food. White flour, white rice, and white bread were created because removing the germ and bran extended shelf life, enabling food to stay "fresh" while traveling from the food factories to the grocery store, sitting on the shelves for days, and then sitting in the home pantry for a week or more without getting moldy or rancid. However, doing so removed most of the fiber, fat, vitamins, and minerals and left only starch, which the body quickly and easily converts to sugar. Dry cereals became popular; they meant less cooking, cleaning, and work and were less expensive. Children preferred processed sugar cereals with a cute little character on the box to good old eggs, bacon, and potatoes. Plus, parents were told that these cereals had all of the essential vitamins and minerals added and were "part of a healthy breakfast." The government began to subsidize certain crops, such as corn and soy, which made them inexpensive. The food industry, looking to save money, started turning cheap corn into cheap and *highly addictive* high-fructose corn syrup, and they added it to everything that they sold. Table sugar became inexpensive, and every family in developed countries is now able to easily afford sugary cereal, cookies, candy, and an ever-growing assortment of toxic, obesity-causing, high-sugar, über-processed "nonfood items" such as Fruit Roll-Ups, cereal bars, pretzels, chips, and energy bars, which are also full of preservatives and artificial colors and flavors. To make matters worse, all of these studies came out correlating dietary fat intake to heart disease and weight gain, so health-care professionals and the US government began to drill the message into our heads that dietary fat should be avoided at all costs. *So the food industry happily responded by creating all of these "fat-free" and "low-fat" "nonfoods" that were actually much worse for us, because they were even more processed; most or all of the fat was removed and replaced with sugar, and we grew even fatter.* Sadly, most children and adults in America now are eating very little real food and living mostly on über-processed nonfoods, full of added sugar, that barely resemble real food, and they don't even realize it. The government knows this, yet it does nothing to stop it, no matter that doing so would certainly cut the cost of health care by preventing the diseases linked with obesity that cheap sugar caused in the first place. Read Michael

Pollan's *In Defense of Food* for a fascinating, detailed, and eye-opening look at the history of the US government's and the American food industry's impact on the Western diet and the disastrous global health consequences of flawed nutritional studies and advice.

The invention of soda further catapulted the country into an obesity epidemic. When we drink calories, such as soda, fruit juice, "vitamin waters," or high-sugar coffee drinks, our bodies do not reduce solid calories to compensate. In other words, liquid calories do not make us feel full and do not signal to our brains that we have just consumed 250 calories; therefore, we continue to eat an average of 250 calories more per day, which can result in significant weight gain—that is, if you only drink one soda per day. It's not only that liquid-sugar drinks add to our caloric intake; they also make us feel hungry, and the high-fructose corn syrup used to sweeten them is turned directly to fat, causing weight gain, high triglycerides, and fatty liver. Diet soda isn't any healthier.

Not only is the food industry making and selling billions of dollars' worth of über-processed crap that they call food, but the portion sizes just keep getting bigger and bigger, and we eat the whole thing because we can't stop. Restaurants are falling over themselves offering bigger portion sizes than their competitors so that we feel like we are getting more for our money. My friend ordered a dish of pasta the other day, and I noticed that the plate they served her contained about six to eight servings of pasta! And that was in a "healthy" restaurant! Eating has become dangerous and deadly, and our perception of how much food we should eat is completely skewed. This is known as "portion distortion."

If you have a hard time saying no to these über-processed, sugar- and flour-containing nonfoods, know that you are not alone. That is the intended outcome—so that you will keep buying them! The food industry literally spends billions of dollars per year marketing and advertising this poison directly to our children! If processed foods and the Western diet are causing an obesity epidemic in typical children, imagine how fast a child with hypothalamic damage will gain weight in this environment! Most of us are basically living in "the Matrix" ;

we don't even realize that we are not eating real food, that the portion sizes we think are normal are actually three to four times the size that our bodies need, or that sugar or artificial sweetener has been put into almost everything that we eat. We must wake up to the fact that there is another way to eat, that calories are most definitely not all created equal, and that, in order to save our children's lives, we will have to step out of the Matrix and eat differently than the rest of our friends, relatives, and most of the country.

The takeaway here is that one of the main keys to successful weight loss and to keeping the weight off for good, especially in children who are obese or have HO, is to *stop buying and eating high-sugar, über-processed, man-made food as much as possible. Definitely do not keep it in your home.* Eat mostly foods that you could grow, hunt, slaughter, or make for yourself if you had to. I cannot emphasize that enough. Our bodies are just not made to ingest foods that are made in a factory and can sit in the pantry or refrigerator for weeks without spoiling. And don't forget: portion size matters, most especially where carbohydrates and sugar are concerned.

Freeing Ourselves from Foods That Make Us Sick and Fat

I was taught by my former mentor, a dietitian who specialized in food addiction before food addiction was even acknowledged as a real type of addiction, to think of all food as belonging to one of two broad categories: "man-made food" and "nature-made food." *Man-made food is anything that man invented. Man-made food is usually made in a factory and can sit in your pantry or refrigerator for weeks without going bad.*

"Nature-made food," in contrast, is made by "Mother Nature" or God— whichever resonates with you. Nature-made foods are what humans and animals were intended to eat. Who knows better what we should be eating, God or man? Once man starts changing what God gave us to eat, we run into trouble. So one of the most important features of the food plan for hypothalamic obesity is that you eat mostly nature-made food

and stay clear of man-made food as much as possible. Another name for man-made foods is processed foods. There are many definitions of processed food, however. When I refer to man-made or processed foods in this book, I am referring mainly to über-processed foods that contain sugar or flour as a main ingredient or to foods that humans have added artificial colors, flavors, or preservatives to in order to improve taste and increase shelf life.

Eliminating man-made food is integral in making this plan work, but it is also the hardest part to commit to doing. However, it does work, and it does get easier. It's tough in the beginning, and you will need your family and friends' support. Getting über-processed, high-sugar, man-made food out of your life is the key to "taming" your child's hyperphagia, decreasing their food cravings, and reaching and maintaining a healthier weight.

Why do man-made/processed foods cause weight gain? Because they are high in sugar, salt, and taste, which increase food cravings, so we eat too much of them! These foods activate the same "reward center" in our brains as cocaine would. No wonder we can't stop eating them!

Think pasta, bread, chips, crackers, "fruit" snacks, dry cereal, and, of course, candy, donuts, and pastries. They are just too tempting, especially for an individual with hypothalamic obesity who feels hungry all the time. How hard is to pass up potato chips or a giant dish of pasta? Almost impossible. How hard is it to stop eating them once you start? *Very.* Now let's ask ourselves the same question about a nature-made carbohydrate like wild rice. How hard is it to pass up a big plate of steaming wild rice? Not too difficult, really. How hard is it to stop eating wild rice once you start? Not hard at all. You see where I am going with this?

If we want to free ourselves from the addictive power that high-sugar, processed food holds over us, the only way to do that is to stop eating it and replace it with food that humans were designed to eat. In other words, real, nature-made food. Rule of thumb: if it grows from the earth or comes from an animal; if no sugar, flour, or chemicals have been added to it; if nothing has been removed from it; or if you could, theoretically, make it yourself (such as cheese or plain yogurt), then it's OK to eat. If it can only be made in a factory or with the help of machinery, or if sugar, flour, or chemicals have been added, then don't eat it, and don't keep it in the house. *It is unrealistic to think that a child, or even, in most cases, an adult, can be successful at weight loss if there are man-made foods in the house. It's like keeping alcohol in the home of an alcoholic and expecting abstinence.*

Clearing Out the Junk from Your Home

Sadly, many of us wouldn't know what to do with "real food," such as butternut squash or quinoa, if our lives depended on it. But you can learn. *If your child has hypothalamic obesity or is becoming obese, and if you want your child to stop gaining weight at a frightening pace, then you must commit to getting all man-made food out of your house.* Even if you choose to allow the occasional desserts and man-made food, definitely do not keep these foods in your home!

So I suspect that most of the food that you currently keep in your pantry will have to go. Really, the only things that you should have in your pantry are coffee, unsweetened hot cereal (such as oatmeal), nuts, seeds, canned beans, broth, spices, dried grains and beans, popcorn kernels, and cooking oils. There should be almost nothing in there that is ready to eat. The only ready-to-eat food should be in the refrigerator. This means that you will have to dedicate much more of your time to cooking, chopping, and cleaning. Also, if there are any nature-made foods that your child frequently binges on, such as grapes or unsweetened peanut butter, then don't keep those foods in your home either. Yes, that means the whole family will have to change the way that it eats. Again, this *must* be a family endeavor, or else it has very little chance of working.

If this sounds way too overwhelming, then I suggest that you take it slow. Make one change at a time. Maybe first you get rid of the dry cereals and switch to hot breakfast for everyone. This will take some time to adjust to, particularly for the parent or older sibling who will be doing the cooking and cleaning! Then, once everyone is used to that, get rid of the high-sugar, processed snack foods only, and start to replace them with nuts, seeds, avocados, small amounts of fruit, animal protein (including cheese), and tons of nonstarchy vegetables. Lastly, get rid of the flour-containing foods, such as bread, pasta, crackers, pretzels, etc., and replace them with 100 percent *intact* whole grains, such as brown/wild rice, quinoa, legumes, and starchy vegetables like sweet potatoes and butternut squash. Doing this slowly will give you time to learn to cook new foods, particularly the natural grains and starchy vegetables, so that you have something new to add each time you take something away. Get back to eating whole, unprocessed, natural food, the way that Mother Nature intended, and you are halfway to solving your child's weight problems and freeing them and the rest of your family from the control that food has had over your lives.

The Connection between Carbohydrates, Insulin, and Weight Gain

When we eat carbohydrates, they are broken down in your mouth, stomach, and small intestines into smaller molecules, one type of which is a sugar called glucose. Glucose is then absorbed from the small intestine into the bloodstream. The bloodstream is like a river; it carries and delivers nutrients from the food we eat to various parts of the body. Our bloodstream carries the glucose to cells all over the body, where it is either converted to energy or sent on "down the river" to be stored for later use. Imagine your cells and your bloodstream are two different compartments or "rooms," with a locked "door" connecting the two. Glucose cannot leave the bloodstream and get inside your cells without a special key to unlock that door. That is the function of a hormone called insulin. Insulin is the key that unlocks the doors to our cells so that glucose can leave the bloodstream, where we don't want it hanging out, and go inside our cells, where it is converted to energy. If we eat more carbohydrates than our cells can process or need, the bloodstream carries the excess glucose to the liver, where it is turned into glycogen, the storage form of sugar. Most glycogen is stored in our muscles, but some is kept in the liver. Once our stores of glycogen are filled to maximum capacity, the remaining carbs are converted to fat.

In an individual with hypothalamic obesity, too much insulin is released as a result of damage to the hypothalamus, so their insulin levels are high even in a fasting state. This hyperinsulinemia causes hunger and weight gain; that extra weight then closes the "keyholes" so the insulin cannot do its job. The result is that glucose cannot exit the bloodstream and enter the cells, so the cells starve because, even though there is plenty of glucose floating around in the blood, it cannot get inside the cells and therefore cannot be used by the body. So the pancreas gets a signal that the insulin it just pumped out is not working, and it pumps out even more insulin to try to fix the problem. This is called insulin resistance. Then, we eat more because more insulin makes us feel hungry, even if we just ate. It becomes a vicious cycle that makes weight loss very, very difficult.

Obese children without HO also develop the vicious cycle of weight gain and insulin resistance; the only difference is that it's not hypothalamic damage that causes it. It's the high-sugar, man-made foods they eat, their sedentary lifestyle, and the subsequent weight gain that cause insulin resistance. Therefore, the key to weight loss and decreased appetite in both groups is to minimize the amount of insulin being pumped out or secreted by the pancreas. There are several ways to do that besides just cutting out processed foods, and we will use all of them.

Carbohydrates are the biggest trigger of insulin secretion. Therefore, the best way to minimize insulin secretion, lose weight, and minimize feelings of hunger (it can be done!), other than eliminating carbs altogether, is to (1) strictly limit your carbohydrate intake, (2) make sure that any carb you eat is naturally high in fiber, (3) space your carbohydrates out evenly throughout the day, and (4) make sure the carbs you choose contain as little sugar and flour as possible. Following one of my food plans will ensure that you are doing all of these things.

Types of Carbs Do Matter

Of the utmost importance in beating this condition, besides limiting carbs, is the *type* of carbs we eat. *Man-made carbs are a recipe for over-eating, increased food cravings, and weight gain—hypothalamic obesity or not. In those with HO, there is no question that consuming man-made carbs exacerbates hyperphagia.* Nature-made carbs, however—especially nonstarchy vegetables but also 100 percent whole, intact, and unrefined grains, starchy vegetables, legumes, and fruit—are naturally designed to slow the digestion process; their high fiber content delays gastric emptying, and it takes more time and effort for our bodies to break them down and convert them to glucose. This slower digestion process slows the rate at which glucose enters the bloodstream, which results in an insulin trickle rather than an insulin surge. Nature-made carbs are also much less likely to trigger food cravings. That doesn't mean you have a free pass to eat as much of them as you like; the amounts of these nature-made carbs need to be controlled and minimized for sure, and you can find the suggested portion sizes in the food plan section of this book.

I realize that cutting out most flour- and sugar-containing food may sound overwhelming if you are used to eating mainly man-made foods, but I promise that by cutting them out, you can "retrain" your taste buds to enjoy nature-made food. Hypothalamic obesity or not, we all benefit from decreasing, or ideally stopping, consumption of man-made, high-sugar carbs. Not only will this result in weight loss but avoiding man-made carbs and replacing them with high-fiber, nature-made carbs decreases inflammation and the risk of heart disease and many types of cancer while improving energy levels, concentration, brain health, immunity (protection from colds and flu), and much more. So when I suggest that the whole family make these changes, it's not only for the benefit of the obese child but for the entire family, even if the others are at a healthy weight already.

Trigger Foods

Food cravings are real and not only for individuals with hypothalamic obesity. I think that most people can identify certain foods that, when eaten, start them on a downward spiral of binge eating or feeling out of control with food. If they avoid these foods, they find it much easier to control their hyperphagia and/or food cravings.

Some individuals with HO report that there are three common groups of foods that trigger or "turn on" their hyperphagia: (1) certain high-sugar fruits or too much fruit in general, (2) foods that contain flour, such as bread, pasta, crackers, etc., and (3) foods that contain sugar, such as candy, baked goods, and processed foods. I have explained the reason that man-made, flour-containing foods and sugar increase cravings already, so now I will discuss fruit.

I certainly can see how certain fruits might increase cravings in some, but not all, individuals with hyperphagia. My son, for example, has to be very careful with grapes and watermelon. He is able to eat all other fruits and is not triggered to eat more by doing so. However, when there are grapes or watermelon in the house, he just cannot stick to his allotted portion size. Therefore, we do not keep these fruits in the house, as they so obviously derail him from his weight-loss efforts.

Trigger foods are different for everyone. You know your child best, and if certain foods cause these issues, then my advice is to completely abstain from eating them and definitely keep them out of the house.

Smart Alternatives to Common Trigger Foods

Trigger Foods (Man-Made Food)	Smart Food (Nature-Made Food) Alternative with Appropriate Serving Size
Pretzels	Popcorn (½ oz.)
Crackers (made with any type of flour)	Mary's Gone Crackers or Flackers (1 oz.)
Potato chips / tortilla chips	Nuts (½–1 oz.), plain plantain chips (1 oz.), roasted seaweed (1 package)
Cereal bars / energy bars	4 oz. sliced apples with 1 tbsp. unsweetened nut butter
Dry cereal with milk	Hot, unsweetened oatmeal (1 oz. dry) with ⅛ tsp. raw honey and 1 packet stevia leaf
Cookies	Celery sticks with 1 tbsp. nut butter and 4 dark chocolate chips or ½ dark chocolate–covered frozen banana
Candy	Dark chocolate chips (5–7)
Fat-free or low-fat salad dressing	1 tbsp. regular salad dressing (less than 1 g sugar per serving) or oil and vinegar
Dried fruit	Pumpkin or sunflower seeds (½–1 oz.)

Smart Alternatives to Common Trigger Foods

Trigger Foods (Man-Made Food)	Smart Food (Nature-Made Food) Alternative with Appropriate Serving Size
Croutons	Sunflower, pumpkin, or hemp seeds (½ oz.)
Pasta	Spaghetti squash, spiralized butternut squash (6 oz.), or spiralized sweet potato or parsnips (3 oz.)
Bread	Lettuce wraps or scooped-out cucumber
High-sugar fruits (such as mangos, grapes, figs, overripe bananas, papaya) IF THEY TRIGGER CRAVINGS	Lower-sugar fruits (berries, yellow bananas, apples, pears, melon, stone fruit)
Fruit juice, soda, sports drinks, or diet soda	Water, unsweetened herbal tea, or water with cucumbers, mint, lemon, etc.
Artificial and nonnutritive sweeteners (aspartame, acesulfame K, sucralose, saccharin, and sugar alcohols)	Stevia, limit 1 packet per day

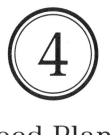

Food Plans

Is the Food Plan for HO Considered Low Carb?

"How many carbs should I eat?"

The answer is not that simple. All human beings are different, and there is actually a spectrum of "carb tolerance," meaning that some people can simply eat more carbs than others without gaining weight. Nutrition is not a one-size-fits-all approach. Carb tolerance varies from person to person depending on activity level, genetics, age, metabolism, weight, height, body composition, insulin sensitivity, body type, and underlying medical conditions, such as diabetes mellitus. I think most of us are waking up to the facts that eating too many carbs leads to obesity and that limiting total carbohydrate intake to some degree is one of the most effective ways to achieve and maintain weight loss. There is no standard definition of a "low-carb diet," and such a diet means different things to different people. Children with hypothalamic obesity have a very low carb tolerance. That means that their bodies cannot process too much carbohydrate at once, and eating too many carbs makes them chronically ill. "Adult-sized" children with HO should not be eating more than 100–150 grams of carbohydrate per day. They may even need less than that—in many cases, much less—in order to achieve weight loss or avoid weight gain, but definitely not more. Children and teens with mild to moderate HO who are not "adult sized" (in terms of their weight or height) require less carbohydrate because they are smaller; thus, their total carbohydrate intake should not exceed 50–120 grams per day, maximum, and again, even that may be too much for some children.

I present two food plans in this book: a "Controlled-Carb Plan" (Food Plan I) and a "Low-Carb Plan" (Food Plan II). The Controlled-Carb Plan strictly limits the amount of carbohydrate *from carbohydrate-dense sources* to 10–20 grams at each meal and each snack. (Carb-dense sources include: starchy vegetables; 100 percent whole, intact grains; fruit; legumes; and unsweetened yogurt). The Controlled-Carb Plan does NOT count carbohydrate from other sources, such as nonstarchy vegetables (veggies that "crunch"), proteins (soy and nuts), and fats (avocado and seeds), because these foods are lower in carbohydrate than carbohydrate-dense foods and also because they contain fiber and/or fat, which slows digestion and thus insulin secretion. Therefore, the total daily carbohydrate will vary daily, depending on your child's protein and fat choices and on how many nonstarchy vegetables they are eating. Even so, the total carbohydrate intake will likely be much lower than your child is used to eating, and it easily resulted in a thirty-pound weight loss in my child.

The Low-Carb Plan (Food Plan II) differs because it limits total carbohydrate intake to *roughly 50–100 grams of carbohydrate per day.* The Low-Carb Plan limits ALL sources of carbohydrate (both carb-dense *and* other sources) to 10–20 grams at each meal and 5–15 grams of carb at each snack and does not allow unlimited nonstarchy vegetables. Therefore, it is a much stricter plan. My son lost an additional ten pounds once we switched to the Low-Carb Plan. Though definitely much lower in carbohydrate than the average American child is used to eating, the Low-Carb Plan (Food Plan II) is not intended to be a ketogenic diet, and it should not induce nutritional ketosis[1]*

---

1. "Nutritional ketosis" is the process of accelerating production of ketones through restriction of dietary carbohydrate.

(if you follow the recommended portion sizes for your child's age). *However, I do recommend checking your child's urine for ketones, and if they are present, please make sure that is OK with your child's doctor. If not, then slowly increase their nonstarchy vegetable or protein intake until ketones are no longer showing up in your child's urine.* You can purchase ketone strips in almost any pharmacy. *Ketones are a byproduct of fat being broken down and used for energy; their presence in the urine of a child (who does not have type 1 diabetes) indicates that the child may be in nutritional ketosis.*

Although I do feel strongly that a modified ketogenic diet (very low carb, moderate protein, and high fat) would be the next step for a child with *severe* HO that is not responsive to a controlled- or low-carb diet, I have not included such a plan in this book. The reason is that I have no experience in using a ketogenic diet at this point. Also, a ketogenic diet causes a loss of sodium and fluid, which has the potential to affect serum sodium levels, which can be dangerous for a child who has diabetes insipidus (DI), especially if they have no thirst mechanism. Therefore, a ketogenic diet should be tried in a child with DI only if they are closely supervised by an endocrinologist knowledgeable in the fluid and electrolyte disturbances that result from nutritional ketosis and a registered dietitian who is experienced in using ketogenic diets in children.

Carbohydrate Counting

Since carbohydrates are the enemy for hypothalamic obesity, it is important for you to learn how to carb count. That means that you need to memorize how many grams of carbohydrate are in standardized portions of nature-made carbohydrates. One "serving" of a carbohydrate-dense food contains roughly 15 grams of carbohydrate, two "servings" of a carb-dense food contains 30 grams of carbohydrate, and so on. The grams of carbohydrate do not refer to the weight of the carbohydrate-containing food but rather to the amount of carbohydrate in the food, which can be confusing. When I talk about the weight of the food or the serving size, I will always use ounces, cups, millimeters, or tablespoons. When I refer to "grams of carb," I am talking about the carb content of the food.

The reason that we must learn to carb count is because for each 12–15 grams[2] of carb that we eat, our blood sugar increases by a certain amount, which then stimulates a certain amount of insulin to be secreted to drive that sugar into our cells. Since the key to weight loss with HO is to minimize insulin secretion, knowing how much carb you are eating is key. *The goal is to eat no more than 10–20 grams of carbohydrate at each meal and 5–15 grams at each snack (depending on which food plan you are following), with a limit of three meals and three carb-containing snacks per day.* Carb counting is a system that is used by people with type 1 diabetes to determine how much insulin they need to give themselves each time they eat. Since we are trying to control our insulin secretion, it makes sense to use the same system.

See the next page for your carb-counting cheat sheet. The following serving sizes will give you 10–20 grams of carbohydrate.

Food Plan Choices

My food plans give you choices of proteins, fat, and carbs. The following lists tell you which foods you may choose from in selecting your proteins, fats, and carbs for the day. You can change it up every day and every meal as you like. I have also listed the portion sizes that provide 10–20 grams of carbohydrate.

---

2.   Generally, one unit of short-acting insulin is required to "dispose of" 12–15 grams of carbohydrate (Diabetes Teaching Center, UCSF).

Carb-Counting Cheat Sheet

Yogurt (unsweetened)	8 oz.
100% intact whole grains	3 oz. cooked
Starchy vegetables	3 oz. cooked (butternut, acorn, and spaghetti squash: 6 oz.)
Fruit	6 oz. (though I suggest not eating more than 4 oz. of fruit for HO)
Legumes	3 oz. cooked
Hot cereal	1 oz. dry
Mary's Gone Crackers	1 oz.
Flackers	1 oz.
Bread	1 slice or 1 oz. (limit to three times a week or fewer)
Nonstarchy vegetables	3 cups raw or 1½ cups cooked

Nature-Made Carb Choices

Food should be weighed *after it has been cooked*, except for hot cereal. An asterisk indicates a "carb-dense" food.

100% Intact Whole Grains*

Serving size listed next to each food = 10–20 g of carbohydrate.

Amaranth (3 oz.)	Millet (3 oz.)	Teff (3 oz.)
Barley (3 oz.)	Oat bran (1 oz. uncooked)	Unsweetened oatmeal (1 oz. uncooked)
Black rice (3 oz.)	Quinoa (3 oz.)	Wheat berries (3 oz.)
Brown rice (3 oz.)	Red rice (3 oz.)	Wild rice (3 oz.)
Bulgur (3 oz.)	Rolled oats (1 oz. uncooked)	
Corn (3 oz.)		
Kasha (3 oz.)		

Starchy Vegetables*

Serving size listed next to each food = 10–20 g of carbohydrate.

Acorn squash (6 oz.)	Jerusalem artichoke (3 oz.)	Rutabaga (6 oz.)
Butternut squash (6 oz.)	Parsnips (3 oz.)	Spaghetti squash (6 oz.)
Cassava, yucca (1½ oz.)	Potatoes (3 oz.)	Taro (1½ oz.)
Celeriac (6 oz.)	Pumpkin (6 oz.)	Yams, sweet potatoes (3 oz.)

Nature-Made Carb Choices

Legumes*

Serving size listed next to each food = 10–20 g of carbohydrate.

Beans (3 oz.) Chickpeas (3 oz.) Edamame (4 oz.)	Green peas (3 oz.) Hummus (3 oz.)	Lentils (3 oz.) Lima Beans (3 oz.)

Yogurt*

12 g of carbohydrate.

Unsweetened, full-fat yogurt (8 oz.)

Fruit*

4 oz. = 10–15 g of carbohydrate.

Avoid dried fruit and high-sugar fruits, such as mangoes, kiwis, grapes, and papaya, as they may trigger cravings for individuals with hyperphagia.

Apples	Clementines	Pineapple
Apricots	Grapefruit	Plums
Avocados	Honeydew	Raspberries
Bananas	Mandarin oranges	Strawberries
Blackberries	Nectarines	Tangelos
Blueberries	Oranges	Tangerines
Cantaloupe	Peaches	Watermelon
Cherries	Pears	

Approved Man-Made Carb Choices

These products, although man made, either do not contain flour or sugar, are very low in carbohydrate and very high in fiber, or have some profound nutritional benefit. Therefore, they are permitted.

Flackers* (1 oz. = 15 g of carb)

Mary's Gone Crackers* (1 oz. = 18 g of carb)

Pasta made from the konjac plant (*Amorphophallus konjac*) (6 oz. = 1 g of carb)

Children following Food Plan I may eat as many nonstarchy vegetables as they like, all day long. This is your tool that you will use to satiate hunger or thoughts of food between meals and snacks. Nonstarchy vegetables do contain some carbohydrate, but you have to eat a lot of them (3 cups raw or 1½ cups cooked) to equal roughly 15 grams of carb. Food Plan II does limit nonstarchy vegetables, unless your child's hyperphagia is severe.

If you or your child does not enjoy raw vegetables, it's fine to sauté them. You can even use a bit of oil, grass-fed butter or ghee, and salt for flavor. It's also fine to add very low-sugar, high-fat salad dressing for dipping or even to melt some parmesan cheese on top.

Nonstarchy vegetables play a huge role in managing hyperphagia. Everywhere we go, I pack **tons of** nonstarchy vegetables. I use the snack-sized Ziploc bags and usually fill three to five of them with sliced bell peppers, jicama, grape or cherry tomatoes, and sliced carrots (these are my son's favorites). You may choose anything from the nonstarchy vegetables list that your children enjoy. JR also loves chopped salads with 1 teaspoon of balsamic dressing and 1 teaspoon of extra-virgin olive oil to snack on. If I have leftover cooked broccoli or zucchini from dinner, I throw that into a container and put it into my purse. I do this before

Nonstarchy Vegetable Choices (Low-Carb)

½ cup cooked or 1 cup raw = ~5 g of carbohydrate.

Only those following the Low-Carb Plan (Food Plan II) need to count carbohydrates from nonstarchy vegetables.

Artichoke	Fennel	Rhubarb
Asparagus	Garlic	Sauerkraut
Beets	Green beans	Scallions
Bok choy	Jicama	Seaweed
Broccoli	Kale	Shallots
Brussels sprouts	Kohlrabi	Snow peas
Cabbage	Leeks	Spinach
Carrots	Lettuce (all varieties)	Sugar snap peas
Cauliflower	Mushrooms	Swiss chard
Celery	Mustard greens	Tomatoes
Collard greens	Okra	Turnips
Cucumbers	Onions	Yellow squash
Dandelion greens	Parsley	Watercress
Eggplant	Peppers	Zucchini
Escarole	Radishes	

we go to birthday parties, movies, restaurants, school, camp, museums, field trips, theme parks, road trips, doctor appointments—everywhere. Doing this prevents fighting and anxiety and decreases the temptation for inappropriate food when he feels hungry. It's so much easier to give him something to eat rather than say, "It's not time to eat now," and face the arguing that would follow. When I say, "Sure. Here are some veggies," he eats them happily and moves on.

But what if my child won't eat vegetables? Simple. When my son complains of hunger between meals and snacks, my reply is always, "You may have nonstarchy vegetables or nothing. Which do you choose?" When he is truly hungry, he eats them. If there is a long time between meals and snacks (more than three hours), I will usually let him have an extra ounce of protein or fat to go with it (usually sliced turkey, avocado, pumpkin or sunflower seeds, or lower-carb nuts such as almonds or walnuts).

I try to put at least two nonstarchy vegetable dishes on the table every night, so that JR can continue to take helpings from those once he has eaten his protein, carb, and fat. I order extra sides of nonstarchy vegetables at restaurants in addition to his meal so that he can fill up on them. I don't really care if they are mixed with bacon, butter, oil, or even salad dressing—as long as it is not "low-fat" dressing. "Low fat" and "fat-free" are code for "high sugar"!

So be proactive. Bring nonstarchy vegetables everywhere you go. This will be one of the main keys to success with both hypothalamic obesity and weight loss in general.

Protein Choices

Proteins marked with an asterisk do contain varying amounts of carbohydrate, but not enough to bother counting unless you are eating more than 1 ounce. The carbohydrate contents of protein and fat choices are listed as a reference for those following the Low-Carb Plan (Food Plan II) *only.*

Animal Protein

Choose organic, 100% grass-fed beef and organic, pasture-raised chicken and eggs whenever possible!

Beef[1]	Poultry (chicken, turkey, duck, hen, pheasant)
Cheese	
Cottage cheese	Pork[2]
Eggs	Ricotta cheese
Fish	Shellfish
Lamb	Wild game (bison, antelope, venison, etc.)
Liver	

1. Lean cuts such as flank or strip steak, sirloin tip, top sirloin steak, eye of round, top round roast and steak, bottom round roast, boneless rump roast, lean stew beef, and 96% lean ground are healthiest, as is 100% grass-fed.

2. Leanest cuts: sirloin roast and chops, cutlets, tenderloin, top loin roast, loin chops, lean and extra-lean ham, canadian bacon, center-cut ham.

Protein Choices

Soy Protein*

Avoid soy "cheese," soy "meats," soy "yogurt," soy "milk,"
or any other man-made, highly processed soy products.
Stick with minimally processed or nature-made soy.

Natto* (1 oz. = 3 grams carbohydrate)

Tempeh* (1 oz. = 3 grams carbohydrate)

Tofu* (1 oz. = 2 grams carbohydrate)

Nut Protein*

Almonds* (1 oz. = 6 g carbohydrate)	Pecans* (1 oz. = 4 g carbohydrate)
Brazil nuts* (1 oz. = 5 g carbohydrate)	Pine nuts* (1 oz. = 4 g carbohydrate)
Hazelnuts* (1 oz. = 5 g carbohydrate)	Walnuts* (1 oz. = 4 g carbohydrate)

High-Carb Nuts*

Weights given are without shell.

Cashews* (1 oz. = 9 g of carbohydrate)	Coconut* (1 oz. = 10 g of carbohydrate)
Chestnuts* (1 oz. = 8 g of carbohydrate)	Pistachios* (1 oz. = 8 g of carbohydrate)

Fat Choices

Serving sizes given are recommended portion sizes.

Avocado* (1 oz. = 3 g of carbohydrate)	Hemp milk* (8 fl. oz. = 2 g of carbohydrate)
Bacon (1 oz.)	Mayonnaise (½ tbsp.)
Butter (1 tsp.)	Oil (all varieties)
Cashew milk (8 fl. oz.)	Olives (1 oz.)
Coconut milk* (no added sugar) (3 oz. = 6 g of carbohydrate)	Salad dressing (1 tbsp.)
	Seeds (hemp, chia, pumpkin, sunflower, flax)* (½ oz. = 3 g of carbohydrate)
Cream cheese (1 tbsp.)	
Ghee (1 tsp.)	Sour cream (2 tbsp.)
Heavy cream (1 tbsp.)	Tahini (½ tbsp.)

Eating Fat Does Not Make You Fat!

Here is the deal: *eating fat does not make us fat.* Remember: eating sugar, man-made food, and too many carbohydrates does. Here is why: *calories are not all created equal.* Fat does not cause insulin to be secreted, which makes it a great choice for weight loss! In addition, fat delays the rate at which the stomach empties. This gives you a feeling of being full. As long as you stick to the recommended portion sizes and total carb intake, and as long as most of the carbs that you do eat are nature-made, high-fiber carbs and your sugar intake remains low, then eating fat will not only help you lose weight but make eating more fun and satisfying.

Heart-healthy, monounsaturated fats are best; however, I am start-ing to question the idea that saturated fat is the demon that it has been made out to be. My experience as a nutritionist has shown me that, *in the context of a low-sugar, nature-made, low(ish)-carb, high-fiber diet,* you can lose weight and lower your risk of heart disease even if you include saturated fat in your diet. JR's lipid levels have all decreased to the normal range, and he lost forty pounds eating yogurt (made with whole milk) and beef one to two times per week and cooking with ghee or butter every day. I couldn't even tell you how much saturated fat JR eats daily, because I don't keep track of it. The amount and types of carbs are my main focus.

Food Plans: Key Points

1. *Eat mostly protein, some healthy fat, and nonstarchy vegetables* at each meal and snack.

2. If following the **Controlled-Carb Plan** (**Food Plan I**), limit carbohydrates to approximately *10–20 grams of nature-made, car-bohydrate-dense foods* at each meal and *10–20 grams at each snack.* Carbohydrates from nonstarchy vegetables, nuts, seeds, avocado, and soy protein are not counted.

3. If following the **Low-Carb Plan** (**Food Plan II**), limit carbohydrates to *10–20 grams of nature-made carbohydrates* at each meal *and 5–15 grams of nature-made carbohydrates* at each snack. Young children (four to six years old) should use the lower end of the portion size ranges given. Older children may start with the higher end and decrease if necessary. Carbohydrate from all sources must be counted if following the Low-Carb Plan. This includes carbohydrates from nuts, seeds, avocado, and soy.

4. *Don't focus on how many grams of fat or how many calories your child is eating.* Focus on feeding them the correct portion sizes and the right

kind of carbohydrates. Purchase a food scale to ensure success and to keep portion sizes from slowly growing over time. Always weigh your food before you eat.

5. *Limit bread to a maximum of three times per week, or cut it out completely.* Some may do better to avoid bread entirely, especially when you first institute the food plan. One slice of bread equals roughly 15 grams of carbohydrate. Don't double up on carbs when you serve bread; rather, replace the carb you usually eat at that meal with one slice of bread.

6. *Limit fruit to two to three servings per day*, 4 ounces maximum per serving.

7. Keep the temptation minimal. *Your child will not succeed with high-temptation, über-processed, man-made food in the house.* Choose your parties, social events, camps, and even schools (if possible) carefully. Avoid buffets.

8. *The whole family must do this together, or it has very little chance of working.* This is a family endeavor. I cannot stress that enough.

9. One dessert per week of three hundred calories or fewer is permitted; *do not choose fat-free or low-fat desserts such as frozen yogurt, jelly beans, or cotton candy.* Some examples of higher-fat desserts that we enjoy once a week are: one scoop of ice cream (*ask for a "child's size"; even a "small" is too big in the United States*), one donut, one small cookie, one brownie, or one slice of birthday cake. Do not keep desserts in your home; rather, go out and eat them. If you suspect that your child may have a sugar or food addiction, or if the once-a-week dessert increases cravings or sneaking, then it would be best to not have a weekly dessert or to try very low-sugar "paleo" desserts instead.

10. Don't eat any food (other than the once-a-week dessert) that has more than 5 grams of sugar per serving. *The less sugar, the better.*

11. *Do not allow your children to drink anything other than water, herbal tea, and the occasional unsweetened nut or hemp milk.* If they don't like the taste of water, then I suggest buying or renting a reverse osmosis water filter or adding some lemon or cucumber slices to your water. *Cutting out all fruit juice, cow's milk, soda, sports drinks, and artificially sweetened beverages is the first thing you should do.* This includes beverages sweetened with stevia leaf. It is OK to use small amounts of fruit juice (in a marinade) or cow's milk (in a frittata) in cooking.

Nutrition intervention must be individualized in order to be successful. We are all unique and have different body types, percent lean body mass, starting weights, and resting metabolism, and we take different medications and have different medical conditions, not to mention varying degrees of hypothalamic damage. Some exercise, and some do not. Some children attend schools that have strict rules prohibiting them from giving children candy and other low-nutrient, high-calorie, processed foods and sugar-containing drinks, and some attend schools where junk food is sold to students by teachers in class. It is impossible for me to write one food plan, or even two, that will work with every child with hypothalamic obesity.

The portion sizes that I recommend in these food plans may need to be adjusted in order to result in weight loss for your child. As I said, no two children are alike. The portion sizes in Food Plan I are based on what resulted in weight loss for my son. Your child may respond very differently depending on their degree of hypothalamic damage, exercise, insulin levels, etc. I suggest you start with the lower end of the suggested ranges of protein and carb and increase only if your child loses more than two pounds per week or if they are too hungry and still sneaking food.

Food Plan I: Controlled-Carb Food Plan for HO

This plan is designed for obese children and teens who have mild to moderate HO, who are constantly complaining of hunger or stealing food (or money to buy food), *and who also weigh at least 150 to 160 pounds.* I have listed some ideas for proteins, fats, and carbs, but feel free to use anything from the protein, fat, and carb lists earlier in the chapter. This is the more liberal carb plan of the two. Remember to limit fruit to two to three servings per day.

Breakfast (6:00–7:30 a.m.)	
Carb	1 oz. (weight uncooked) unsweetened oatmeal or oat bran **OR** 3 oz. grain/ starchy vegetable/legume **OR** 8 oz. unsweetened yogurt **OR** 4 oz. fruit
Fat	1 tsp. oil or butter or ghee (if needed to cook)
Protein	1–2 oz. animal or soy protein **OR** ½–1 oz. nut protein
Vegetable	Nonstarchy only, no limit
"Between-Snack" Snack (optional)	
Vegetable	Nonstarchy only, no limit
Morning Snack (9:00–10:30 a.m.)	
Carb	4 oz. fruit **OR** ½ oz. popcorn **OR** 8 oz. unsweetened yogurt
Fat or Protein	1–2 oz. animal or soy protein **OR** ½–1 oz. nut protein **OR** 1–2 oz. avocado **OR** ½ oz. seeds
Vegetable	*Optional.* Nonstarchy only, no limit
"Between-Snack" Snack (optional)	
Vegetable	Nonstarchy only, no limit
Lunch (11:30 a.m.–12:30 p.m.)	
Carb	3 oz. cooked grain or starchy vegetable or legume **OR** 4 oz. fruit
Fat	1 tsp. oil or butter or ghee **OR** ½–1 tbsp. regular salad dressing **OR** ½ oz. seeds **OR** 1 oz. avocado
Protein	3–4 oz. animal or soy protein
Vegetable	Nonstarchy only, no limit

"Between-Snack" Snack (optional)	
Vegetable	Nonstarchy only, no limit

Afternoon Snack (2:30–3:30 p.m.)	
Carb	4 oz. fruit **OR** ½ oz. popcorn **OR** 8 oz. unsweetened yogurt
Fat or Protein	1–2 oz. animal *or* soy protein **OR** ½–1 oz. nut protein **OR** 1–2 oz. avocado **OR** ½ oz. seeds
Vegetable	*Optional.* Nonstarchy only, no limit

"Between-Snack" Snack (optional)	
Protein	*Only if necessary.* 1–2 oz. animal protein **OR** ½–1 oz. nut protein
Vegetable	Nonstarchy only, no limit

Dinner (5:00–7:00 p.m.)	
Carb	3 oz. whole grain *or* starchy vegetable *or* legume **OR** 4 oz. fruit
Fat	1 tsp. oil *or* butter *or* ghee **OR** 1 tbsp. regular salad dressing
Protein	3–4 oz. animal *or* soy protein
Vegetable	Nonstarchy only, no limit

"Between-Snack" Snack (optional)	
Vegetable	Nonstarchy only, no limit

Evening Snack (7:00–9:00 p.m.)	
Fat or Protein	1–2 oz. (cooked) animal *or* soy protein **OR** ½ oz. nut protein **OR** 1–2 oz. avocado **OR** ½ oz. seeds
Vegetable	Nonstarchy only, no limit

Why Aren't We Fighting Anymore?

I think it is important to understand why JR and I have gone from fighting over food several times a day to arguing maybe once a month.

Before we started this food plan, I weighed and measured all of my son's food, and almost all foods were permitted, although processed and sugary foods were discouraged. This was a "NO!" food plan. "Eating time is over." "You cannot eat right now. You have to wait an hour." "NO, you cannot have more than half a cup of pretzels." "No, that is too much." "You can only have one bowl of cereal a day, not three!" Children with hypothalamic obesity are hungry all of the time. Telling them, "No, you cannot eat now," is beyond upsetting for them and results in all sorts of control battles for parents and behavioral problems for these kids.

Food Plan I is more of a "YES!" plan. Now, when my son is hungry between meals, instead of hearing, "No!" he hears, "Yes! You may eat! You may have as many nonstarchy vegetables as you like!" And not just raw vegetables, but delicious seasoned, roasted, or sautéed vegetables. Still hungry? "OK, have a little extra protein or healthy fat, since dinner will be later this evening."

I am no longer asking him to ignore his hunger or to fight it. The Carb-Controlled Food Plan for HO satisfies his frequent hunger and decreases his cravings and drive to overeat. Since he knows that he can have nonstarchy vegetables anytime he likes and as much as he likes, he no longer feels anxious or like he has to shove as much food into his mouth on the sly as possible because he won't be allowed to eat later. The drive to sneak food has dramatically decreased.

Food Plan II: Low-Carb Food Plan
(50-100 Grams of Carbohydrate)

Food Plan II is for younger children with hypothalamic obesity, children and teens with HO who weigh fewer than 140 to 150 pounds, obese children and teens who have hypothalamic obesity *without hyperphagia*, and children and teens with hypothalamic obesity who do not see results (weight loss or cessation of weight gain) following Food Plan I. *Very young children should use the lowest end of the serving size ranges given and increase as needed. Older or heavier children should start with the higher end and decrease if necessary.* You will need to experiment with which serving size works for your child.

Nonstarchy vegetables are permitted between snacks and meals *only if necessary*. This will slightly increase carbohydrate intake.

One high-fat, portion-controlled dessert of three hundred calories or fewer may be eaten once a week. This should be done only if doing so does not trigger cravings or cause bingeing or tantrums. Examples include: *a child's size* (not a "small," due to portion distortion) serving or a single scoop of full-fat ice cream, one thin slice of cake, one chocolate chip cookie (no larger than the palm of your child's hand), or one donut (the size of your child's palm). Very small "special treats" can be given two to three times per week, such as five to seven dark chocolate chips, a very small lollipop, a very small piece of candy, etc. If eating "real" desserts causes problems (increased cravings, food stealing, etc.), then try a low-sugar / low-carb "paleo-type dessert."

Breakfast (6:00–7:00 a.m., ~10–20 g of carbohydrate)	
Carb	1 oz. high-carb nut **OR** ½ oz. unsweetened oatmeal *or* oat bran **OR** 1–2 oz. grain/starchy vegetable *or* legume **OR** 4 oz. unsweetened yogurt **OR** 2–3 oz. fruit
Fat	1 tsp. butter *or* ghee *or* oil (if needed to cook) **OR** ½ oz. seeds **OR** 1 slice bacon
Protein	1–2 oz. animal *or* soy protein **OR** ½–1 oz. nut protein
Vegetable	Nonstarchy only, ½ cup cooked **OR** 1 cup raw
Morning Snack (9:30–10:00 a.m.; ~5–15 g of carbohydrate)	
Carb	½–1 oz. high-carb nut **OR** 2 oz. avocado **OR** 2–3 oz. fruit **OR** ½ oz. popcorn **OR** 4 oz. unsweetened yogurt **OR** ½ cup cooked (*or* 1 cup raw) nonstarchy vegetables
Protein	1–2 oz. animal **OR** ½–1 oz. nut protein
Lunch (11:30 a.m.–12:30 p.m.; ~10–20 g of carbohydrate)	
Carb	1 oz. high-carb nut **OR** 1–2 oz. grain *or* starchy vegetable *or* legume **OR** 2–3 oz. fruit
Fat	1 tsp. butter *or* ghee *or* oil *or* ½–1 tbsp. regular salad dressing
Protein	1–4 oz. animal protein
Vegetable	Nonstarchy only, ½ cup cooked **OR** 1 cup raw

Afternoon Snack (2:30–3:30 p.m.; ~5–15 g of carbohydrate)	
Carb	½–1 oz. high-carb nut **OR** 2 oz. avocado **OR** 2–3 oz. fruit **OR** ½ oz. popcorn **OR** 4 oz. unsweetened yogurt **OR** ½ cup cooked **OR** 1 cup raw nonstarchy vegetables
Protein	1–2 oz. animal **OR** ½–1 oz. nut protein
Dinner (5:00–7:00 p.m.; ~10–20 g of carbohydrate)	
Carb	1 oz. high-carb nut **OR** 1–2 oz. grain *or* starchy vegetable *or* legume **OR** 2–3 oz. fruit
Fat	1 tsp. butter *or* ghee *or* oil
Protein	1–4 oz. animal **OR** ½–1 oz. nut protein
Vegetable	Nonstarchy only, ½ cup cooked **OR** 1 cup raw
Evening Snack (7:00–9:00 p.m.; ~5–10 g of carbohydrate)	
Protein	1–2 oz. animal **OR** ½–1 oz. nut protein
Vegetable	Nonstarchy only, ½ cup cooked **OR** 1 cup raw

The "Non-Food Plan" Plan

This really is not a food plan. It's a general way of eating for people who feel overwhelmed at the idea of weighing and measuring all of their child's food or counting carbs. It's also the way we eat at restaurants or at parties. We don't bring a food scale with us; rather, we just make sure that most of the foods that we order are proteins, fats, and nonstarchy vegetables and that only a very small amount is carbohydrates (mostly, but not always, nature made). So, for example, at a restaurant, JR might order chicken, steak, or fish; a salad with some berries, pecans, and cheese sprinkled on it; and a side (or several) of nonstarchy vegetables; and we might all share an appetizer like stuffed mushrooms, a shrimp cocktail, an avocado cucumber salad, or perhaps a bowl of tortilla soup filled with chicken and vegetables or a very small corn tamale *or* a small portion of fried plantains.

> Create a line graph that shows your child's weekly weights, and tape it to the refrigerator or pantry. That way, they can see how the way they are eating and exercising affects their weight. This was incredibly motivating for our son!

A family who follows the "Non–Food Plan" plan might make something like scrambled eggs, sausage, and a small serving of fruit for breakfast; a handful of nuts and steamed broccoli with melted cheese for a snack; and a salad with a good amount of chicken, avocado, and salad dressing, a small amount of edamame or garbanzo beans, and some celery sticks with peanut butter for lunch. Dinner might be fish tacos with one very small corn tortilla, jicama slaw, and guacamole and roasted nonstarchy vegetables, or it could be spaghetti squash with meat sauce and grilled eggplant. The evening snack might be a few slices of turkey with sunflower seeds and cherry tomatoes.

Just be sure to switch to weighing at least the carbs if your child's carb portion sizes start to become bigger and bigger and become a point of contention between you and your child.

If this sounds like the plan for you, then become familiar with the list of approved nature-made carbohydrates so that you know which foods should comprise the smallest amount of your child's diet. *Disclaimer: This way of eating cannot ensure that your child is eating enough carbohydrates to avoid nutritional ketosis, so be sure to check their urine for ketones (you can purchase ketone strips in any pharmacy). If they are present, discuss this with your child's doctor. If necessary, slowly increase the amount of carbohydrates your child is eating until there are no ketones in their urine.*

	Breakfast	Snack	Lunch
Monday	1 egg omelet with 1 oz. parmesan cheese 1 oz. plain oatmeal (⅛ tsp. raw honey with 1 packet stevia)	1 tbsp. unsweetened nut butter on celery sticks 4 oz. blueberries	4 oz. chicken or chicken salad (with mayo) Salad with ½ oz. sunflower seeds, 3 oz. corn, and 1 tbsp. balsamic dressing
Tuesday	1–2 oz. turkey sausage 4 oz. fruit	1 oz. sunflower seeds 4 oz. sliced apples	2 oz. roast beef, rolled up 2 oz. cheddar cheese 3 oz. potato salad (with mayo) Cucumber tomato salad with 1 tsp. balsamic and 2 tsp. olive oil
Wednesday	1–2 scrambled eggs 3 oz. breakfast potatoes with sautéed onions and bell peppers	2 oz. chicken salad with mayo 4 oz. strawberries	2 oz. mozzarella cheese balls 2 oz. prosciutto 4 oz. watermelon Sliced tomatoes Grilled or roasted nonstarchy vegetables *All of the above drizzled with 1 tsp. balsamic vinegar and 1 tsp. olive oil

Snack	Dinner	Snack
4 oz. pineapple 2 oz. sliced ham or turkey	4 oz. sliced chicken breast (cooked any style) on salad with ¼ cup green peas and 1 tbsp. salad dressing, grape tomatoes, bell peppers, jicama, and cucumbers	½–1 oz. nuts Spinach salad
1 oz. sliced turkey ¼ cup hummus Jicama or carrot slices 2 oz. clementine orange	4 oz. wild salmon or halibut 3 oz. quinoa Grilled or roasted nonstarchy vegetables	1–2 oz. chicken or tuna salad Sliced carrots
10 Mary's Gone Crackers "nachos" with 1 oz. melted cheese and 1 oz. avocado	4 oz. sautéed shrimp 3 oz. brown rice Zucchini "zoodles" sautéed with 1 tsp. ghee or canola oil	1 oz. pumpkin seeds Sliced bell peppers

	Breakfast	Snack	Lunch
Thursday	1 oz. almonds 4 oz. fruit smoothie	2 oz. turkey or ham ½ oz. popcorn	4 oz. sautéed shrimp 3 oz. brown rice Zucchini noodles ("zoodles") 1 oz. avocado drizzled with 1 tsp. olive oil and 1 tsp. white-wine vinegar
Friday	1 slice 100% whole-grain toast 1 egg omelet with 1 oz. swiss cheese 1 oz. avocado Sliced bell pepper	1 oz. pistachios (no shell) 4 oz. cantaloupe	4 oz. egg, turkey bacon, and cheese frittata 3 oz. roasted sweet potato wedges Green beans
Saturday	¼–½ cup cottage or ricotta cheese (whole milk) 4 oz. berries	1–2 hard-boiled egg salad (with 1 tsp. mayo and mustard) 10 Mary's Gone Crackers	4 oz. turkey sausage 6 oz. spaghetti squash Roasted cauliflower with paprika, sprinkled with melted parmesan cheese
Sunday	2 oz. turkey bacon 1 oz. unsweetened oatmeal (⅛ tsp. raw honey with 1 packet stevia)	1 oz. chocolate paleo granola 3 oz. sliced apples	4 oz. tuna salad with 1 tbsp. mayo 3 oz. brown rice Chopped veggie salad with 1 oz. avocado 1 tbsp. low-sugar dressing

Snack	Dinner	Snack
4 oz. blueberries ½ oz. almonds	4 oz. egg, turkey bacon, and cheese frittata 3 oz. roasted sweet potato wedges Sautéed green beans with mushrooms	1–2 oz. turkey or ham Sliced jicama sticks
4 oz. strawberries 1–2 oz. turkey or ham	4 oz. turkey sausage 6 oz. spaghetti squash, roasted eggplant, and ½ cup marinara sauce	1 tbsp. unsweetened nut butter Cherry tomatoes
4 oz. watermelon 2 oz. mozzarella cheese Drizzle with 1 tsp. balsamic and 1 tsp. olive oil	Eat out	1 oz. sausage Sautéed zucchini slices
8 oz. milk (soy, hemp, or flax) 1 tbsp. almond butter	4 oz. grilled sirloin steak 3 oz. baked parsnip or potato french fries Roasted brussels sprouts	1 oz. turkey or ham Broccoli with 1 oz. cheese

	Breakfast	Snack	Lunch
Monday	1 scrambled egg 1 oz. turkey sausage 1 oz. oatmeal with ⅛ tsp. raw honey and 1 packet stevia Carrot sticks	1–2 oz. colby cheese stick ½ oz. popcorn	Mini pizza (made with whole-wheat One Bun) with 2 oz. mozzarella cheese and tomato sauce 2 oz. sliced pepperoni Sliced cucumbers with 1 tbsp. ranch dressing
Tuesday	1 tbsp. unsweetened nut butter 1 slice 100% whole-grain toast Sliced jicama	4 oz. clementine oranges ½ oz. cashews	2–3 oz. meatballs 3 oz. brown rice or 3 oz. spiralized sweet potatoes with marinara sauce Steamed broccoli with 1 oz. melted cheese
Wednesday	4 oz. unsweetened plain yogurt with 2 oz. blueberries or strawberries and ½ oz. hemp/chia seeds mixed in	4 oz. pear slices 1–2 oz. turkey or ham	Grilled cheese sandwich with One Bun (or similar) bread, made with 2 oz. cheddar cheese 1–2 oz. rolled turkey, salad with 1 tbsp. ranch dressing

Snack	Dinner	Snack
1–2 hard-boiled eggs 1–2 tsp. ranch dressing 4 oz. strawberries	2–3 oz. meatballs (90–95% lean, grass-fed beef/bison) or meat sauce 3 oz. brown rice or 3 oz. spiralized sweet potatoes with ½ cup marinara sauce Steamed broccoli with 1 oz. melted cheese	1 oz. cheese Steamed broccoli
1–2 oz. turkey 1 oz. popcorn	3–4 oz. fish sticks 3 oz. quinoa Grilled or roasted carrots Vegetables drizzled with 1 tsp. olive oil	½–1 oz. mixed nuts Grilled or roasted carrots
1 oz. colby cheese cubes +/- 1 oz. pepperoni 4 oz. sliced apples	3–4 oz. sliced ham with 1 oz. cubed pineapple kebabs 2 oz. brown rice Sliced bell peppers	1 oz. turkey or ham Sliced bell peppers

	Breakfast	Snack	Lunch
Thursday	1 egg, any style +/- 1 oz. cheese 3 oz. breakfast potatoes	1 oz. turkey or ham ¼ cup hummus Jicama or carrot slices 2 oz. clementine orange	3–4 oz. sliced ham with 1 oz. cubed pineapple kebabs 2 oz. brown rice Sliced bell peppers
Friday	1 tbsp. unsweetened nut butter 4 oz. sliced apples or pears Sliced bell peppers	10 Mary's Gone Crackers "nachos" with 1–2 oz. melted cheese	3–4 oz. turkey sausage with mustard 3 oz. baked french fries Sugar snap peas
Saturday	1 scrambled egg 1 tsp. grass-fed butter 1 oz. turkey sausage links 1 oz. oatmeal with ⅛ tsp. honey and 1 packet stevia Carrot sticks	4 oz. blueberries ½ oz. almonds	2 oz. mozzarella cheese balls 1–2 oz. sliced ham Sliced tomatoes drizzled with balsamic vinegar and olive oil Roasted cauliflower
Sunday	6 oz. unsweetened yogurt 1 oz. blueberries or strawberries ½ oz. hemp/chia seeds mixed in	4 oz. fruit smoothie 1–2 oz. turkey or ham	2 oz. roast beef, rolled up 1–2 oz. swiss cheese, rolled up 3 oz. potato salad with ½ tbsp. mayo Mini pickles

Snack	Dinner	Snack
4 oz. unsweetened yogurt ½ oz. hemp/chia seeds mixed 1–2 oz. berries	3–4 oz. turkey sausage with mustard 3 oz. baked french fries Cherry tomatoes	½ cup cottage or ricotta cheese with cinnamon Sliced carrots
1–2 oz. roast beef 10 Mary's Gone Crackers Whole-grain mustard	2–3 oz. turkey or all-beef hot dog (no nitrites) with 1 oz. cubed cheddar cheese Kebabs Corn on the cob (½ cob) Sliced carrot sticks	1–2 oz. hot dog (no nitrates/nitrites) Sliced jicama sticks
1–2 oz. string cheese 4 oz. watermelon	3–4 oz. hamburger with 3 oz. baked potato or parsnip french fries Cherry tomatoes	1 tbsp. unsweetened nut butter Cherry tomatoes ½–1 oz. nuts
4 oz. pear slices 1–2 oz. turkey or ham	Eat out	1–2 oz. cheese Sliced carrots

	Breakfast	Snack	Lunch
Monday	1–2 oz. turkey sausage ½ oz. plain oatmeal with ⅛ tsp. honey and 1 packet stevia	1–2 oz. fresh mozzarella cheese balls with cherry tomatoes and 2 oz. avocado	1–4 oz. chicken salad with ½ oz. sunflower seeds 2–3 oz. fruit or 1 cup salad (lettuce with tomatoes, cucumbers, and 1 tbsp. salad dressing)
Tuesday	1–2 oz. scrambled eggs 1–2 oz. hash browns	1–2 oz. any cheese 2–3 oz. mixed raspberries and blackberries	Mini pizza (made with whole-wheat One Bun) with 1–2 oz. mozzarella cheese and tomato sauce 1–2 oz. sliced pepperoni 1 cup cucumbers with 1 tbsp. ranch dressing
Wednesday	1–2 oz. pork sausage 2–3 oz. fruit	1–2 oz. turkey 2 oz. avocado or ½ oz. seeds	1–3 oz. meatballs 1–2 oz. brown rice with marinara sauce 1 cup steamed broccoli with 1 oz. melted cheese

Snack	Dinner	Snack
½–1 oz. almonds with 2–3 oz. berries	1–3 oz. meatballs (90–95% lean, grass-fed beef/bison) or meat sauce 1–2 oz. brown rice or 1–2 oz. spiralized sweet potatoes with ½ cup marinara sauce 1 cup steamed broccoli with 1 oz. melted cheese	1–2 oz. cheese ½ cup steamed broccoli
1–2 oz. turkey with 2–3 oz. melon	1–4 oz. chicken fingers (baked or panfried and breaded with ground pistachios, flaxseed, and parmesan cheese) 1–2 oz. quinoa 1 cup grilled or roasted carrots Vegetables drizzled with 1 tsp. olive oil	½–1 oz. mixed nuts 1 cup cucumber slices
½–1 oz. cashews with 1–2 oz. sliced chicken	1–4 oz. pork or turkey loin with 1 oz. cubed pineapple kebabs 1–2 oz. mashed sweet potato ½ cup sugar snap peas	1–2 oz. turkey or ham 4 oz. sliced carrots

	Breakfast	Snack	Lunch
Thursday	1 egg omelet with 1 oz. cheese 1–2 oz. black beans 1 oz. avocado Salsa	1 string cheese stick ½ oz. popcorn	Grilled cheese tuna melt sandwich with One Bun (or similar) bread, made with ½–2 oz. cheddar cheese ½–2 oz. tuna salad 1 cup salad with 1 tbsp. ranch dressing
Friday	½ cup ricotta or cottage cheese 2–3 oz. fruit	1–2 oz. thin sliced ham 2–3 oz. pineapple	1–4 oz. sliced ham with 2–3 oz. cubed pineapple kebabs 1 cup sliced bell peppers
Saturday	1–2 oz. turkey bacon ½ oz. plain oatmeal with ⅛ tsp. honey and 1 packet stevia	1–2 oz. chicken salad 2–3 oz. strawberries	1–4 oz. turkey sausage with mustard 1–2 oz. baked french fries 1 cup salad with balsamic and olive oil dressing
Sunday	1 oz. bacon 1 egg omelet 1–2 oz. hash browns	1–2 hard-boiled eggs 2–3 oz. sliced apples	1–4 oz. mozzarella cheese balls with 1 oz. cashews Sliced tomatoes drizzled with balsamic vinegar and olive oil ½ cup grilled or roasted vegetables

Snack	Dinner	Snack
1 tbsp. nut butter on celery with 3 dark chocolate chips and ½ oz. popcorn	1–4 oz. turkey sausage with mustard 1–2 oz. baked french fries ½ cup roasted cauliflower with sprinkle of parmesan cheese	¼–½ cup cottage/ricotta cheese 4 oz. sliced bell peppers
½–1 oz. walnuts with 2–3 oz. clementines	1–3 oz. chicken or all-beef hot dog (no nitrites) with 1 oz. cubed cheddar cheese kebabs Corn on the cob (½ cob) 1 cup sliced carrot sticks	1–2 oz. sliced hot dog (no nitrates/nitrites) 1 cup sliced jicama sticks
1–2 oz. turkey bacon 2 oz. avocado	1–3 oz. hamburger (meat only) topped with 1 slice bacon 2 spaghetti squash fritters ½ cup grilled zucchini	1–2 oz. cheese stick 1 cup cherry tomatoes
2–3 oz. sliced plums 4 oz. yogurt	Eat out	1 oz. sliced ham 1 oz. cheese ½ cup sautéed sugar snap peas

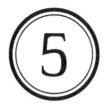

Tips, Ideas, Helpful Hints, and Troubleshooting

More Low-Carb Breakfast Ideas

- 1 oz. pumpkin seeds with 4 oz. unsweetened yogurt
- ½ oz. nut butter with 2–4 oz. banana and 1 oz. turkey sausage
- 1–2 oz. cheese cubes with 2–4 oz. strawberries and ½ oz. sunflower seeds
- 1 mini egg frittata cooked with 1 cup cooked broccoli with 1 oz. melted cheese
- ¼–½ cup ricotta/cottage cheese with 2–4 oz. berries and ½–1 oz. nuts/seeds
- 1–2 oz. sliced turkey or ham with 2–4 oz. fruit
- 1–2 hard-boiled eggs with 2–4 oz. clementines
- 2–4 oz. fruit smoothie or frozen fruit smoothie popsicle with 2 eggs any style
- 2 egg veggie omelet with 2 oz. avocado and 1 oz. black beans
- ½ oz. hot oat bran with ¼ cup whole milk cottage/ricotta cheese and cinnamon with 2 oz. berries

More Snack Ideas

So what are some healthy nature-made snacks that you can feed your children? Here are some of our favorites! Again, adjust servings to match the meal plan you are following.

- Pear slices and celery sticks with almond butter
- Almonds and melon
- Scrambled eggs with cheese and fruit
- Nuts, sunflower seeds, and/or pumpkin seeds with unsweetened greek yogurt
- Apples slices and cheddar cheese
- Banana slices or fried plantains with 1 tablespoon of almond butter
- Cucumber salad with avocado, jicama, grape tomatoes, olive oil, and balsamic vinegar
- Pineapple and ham or turkey kebobs
- Chicken sausage with fruit smoothie
- Baked sweet potato crisps with guacamole
- Mozzarella cheese balls with avocado and tomato salad
- Cottage cheese with cinnamon and fruit
- Sliced bell peppers with hummus and sliced turkey or ham
- Apple slices with almond butter "sandwich"
- Chicken salad with popcorn

Weekly Treat Ideas (Both Food Plans)

- Fruit kebab drizzled with melted dark chocolate
- 1 tablespoon of dark chocolate chips
- Dark chocolate–covered strawberries or bananas
- *Mini / kid's-sized* ice cream scoop
- Frozen dark chocolate–covered banana slices rolled in chopped peanuts
- Dark chocolate chips (1 tablespoon or less) with 2 ounces of raspberries or strawberries

Smart Restaurant Choices

Some of the foods on this list do contain bread crumbs or flour, which is fine if you eat out only once a week. You may be surprised that I have included some fried foods on this list. They are actually lower in carbs than you might think. Rule of thumb: keep the carb portion very small, and eat mostly protein, fat, and nonstarchy vegetables at restaurants.

Smart Restaurant Choices	
American	
Seafood (shrimp, crab, fish fillet, fried calamari, grilled calamari, scallops, lobster, etc.) Potatoes Steak Chicken Corn Vegetables	Quinoa Beans/lentils Brown rice Wild rice Potato leek soup Butternut squash soup
Asian	
Kimchi Lettuce wraps Fresh summer rolls wrapped in rice paper Edamame	Satay (chicken, pork, beef) Sashimi Stir-fried protein with vegetables Brown rice, black rice, red rice

Smart Restaurant Choices

Barbecue

Brisket	Green beans
Pulled chicken or pork	Corn
Turkey	Potato salad
Sausage	

Deli

Nova/lox	Chopped liver
Whitefish	Stuffed cabbage
Sturgeon	Gefilte fish
Herring	Hash browns
Tuna salad	Potatoes
Brisket	Beets / beet soup
Roasted turkey	Vegetables
Roasted chicken	Chicken barley soup
Egg salad	Chicken broth

Mediterranean / Middle Eastern

Grilled calamari	Shakshuka
Souvlakis/kebabs/shish	Shepherd's salad
Tabouleh	Lentil soup
Baba ghanoush	Hummus
Falafel	

Smart Restaurant Choices

Latin American / Spanish

Ceviche	Any seafood tapas or entrée without rice or bread
Any fish/seafood entrée	
Chicken or steak fajitas or tacos (1–2 small corn tortillas maximum)	Any meat/chicken/seafood "a la plancha" or "a la parrilla"
Guacamole	Fried plantains ("maduros" or "tostones")
Tortilla española	Beans
Chorizo (sausage)	Ropa vieja
Jamón serrano (serrano ham)	Pollo guisado
Pisto	Lechón
Patatas bravas (fried potatoes)	Yuca
Gambas al ajillo (garlic shrimp)	Soups
	Olives

Italian

Buffalo mozzarella caprese	Chicken marsala
Carpaccio	Chicken piccata
Prosciutto	Osso buco
Grilled calamari	Shrimp scampi
Fried calamari	Italian salad
Mussels	Olives
Any fish entrée	

What If My Child Won't Eat Nature-Made Food?

I know what many of you are thinking: "My child won't eat like this! It is totally unrealistic to think that my child will accept spaghetti squash instead of pasta." That depends. If your child won't eat nature-made carbs, ask yourself, "Why not?" Is it because their mom, dad, sister, and brother don't eat them? Is it because they say they don't like them? Why aren't they willing to eat nonstarchy vegetables? I don't care if you have to add cheese, ranch dressing, oil and vinegar, or bacon or if you have to mix them in with the protein or nature-made carbs. Just start incorporating nonstarchy vegetables into their lives. That must start with the parents eating nature-made carbs and vegetables. If the parents are unwilling to make some major changes in their own diets, then you are right—this won't work. *This only works if the family does it together.* Parents must model the behavior that they wish their child to emulate or even entertain. Hypothalamic obesity is a condition that negatively affects every single member of the nuclear and extended family, and everyone must be on board to turn things around and make it less of a problem for everyone. If you don't have time to cook, use frozen or raw nonstarchy vegetables and salads or buy nature-made carbs already prepared. It's well worth the money.

Are you hesitating to buy nonstarchy vegetables and nature-made carbs because they are more expensive than processed foods? Consider that insulin injections, diabetes medications, special shoes for diabetic neuropathy, blindness, dialysis, doctor bills, and hospital fees are expensive too, and if you don't stop buying and feeding your children processed, man-made foods, you may soon be forced to pay for those things instead. The cost of vegetables and healthy food is nothing compared to a lifetime of additional pharmaceuticals, doctors, and hospital fees associated with obesity.

Is it because they are always given a choice to eat something different? That brings me to my next point: whether or not your child likes or is willing to eat nonstarchy vegetables, they are the only foods that should be allowed between meals and snacks. If your child complains, the response should be, "Your choice is nonstarchy vegetables or noth-ing. You may have as many as you like." You can sauté them or eat them raw and pair them with dressing, butter, or oil. My son would never have chosen to eat nonstarchy vegetables if I had given him a choice to eat something else.

Ideas to Make Cooking Easier

I realize that this food plan requires a lot of cooking, chopping, and shopping, and you may be asking yourself how you are going to do it. I have a couple of ideas to make things easier.

1. Make at least one extra serving of dinner, and pack the extra serving for your child's lunch the next day. Pack up lunch as you are clean-ing up from dinner so that you don't have to do it in the morning.

2. If you have a babysitter, housekeeper, or older child, assign them the job of chopping and prepping everything you will need to make dinner that night.

3. Make one, two, or three weekly dinner menu plans. Monday nights are always the same meal; Tuesday nights are always the same; etc. This makes the shopping easier and takes the stress out of figuring out what to make for dinner each night. One night a week can be takeout or a dine-in restaurant. One night can be leftovers for the kids while the parent or parents go out to eat.

4. If you don't have time to cook and shop, I highly recommend trying a meal-kit delivery service or personal chef service.

5. Teach your children to help with food prep. Give everyone a job. Distribute the work. If you have a spouse who is able and willing to help out with cooking and/or cleaning, then take advantage.

Meal Delivery Services

What's a working mom or single parent to do? Working moms and single parents have to do it all. Every morning, they get the kids fed and dressed and delivered to school on time (on a good day), put in a full day's work, go to the grocery store several times a week, pick up their children from school, drive children to after-school activities, and then go home and get homework done, make dinner, clean up afterward, and make lunches for the next day! It's admirable what working moms and single parents do on a daily basis, and, understandably, healthy cooking may get left out. If this sounds like your life, and if you don't have time to do the cooking necessary to improve your child's health, then I urge you to consider trying a meal-kit delivery service or even a personal chef. Sounds crazy, right? Too expensive? Maybe not. Let's look at each individually.

When to Consider a Personal Chef

For the first year and a half during the time it took JR to lose forty pounds, I cooked or prepared every meal and snack, a minimum of six times per day. I went to the grocery store almost every day (because I am unorganized) and spent a fortune on mostly organic whole foods. Most of my day was: shop, chop, cook, clean, repeat. It was worth it to save my child's life and improve the entire family's health, but it sure wasn't easy. How on earth is a mom who works full time or a single parent going to do all of this?

OK, I have a confession to make. When I got the idea to write this book, things fell into place much faster than I had expected. I met with a publisher, thinking I'd have to meet with several before one agreed to take me on. The exact opposite happened. I met with a publisher who loved my book idea and gave me a two- to four-month deadline in which to get it written. Yikes! Did I mention that it was summertime, the kids were out of school, and I was running around with them all day? I was extremely stressed out about how I was going to do it all.

My Ayurveda practitioner told me that I'd have to get help with the cooking. She suggested hiring a personal chef. What? Was she crazy? Who does that? Celebrities, perhaps, but not me!

"Do some research, and look at the numbers," she advised. So I did. I did a Google search and found a local, health-conscious company that cooked mostly organic food in their own kitchen and would deliver a week's worth of family dinners to my home once a week. They catered to a wide variety of diets and food allergies. I explained the way that we eat, and they were able to accommodate. She gave me weekly price for the chef's fee and said I would also pay for groceries and delivery.

So I decided to try it for one week. I calculated how much money I spent per week at the grocery store on meal-prep items and compared it to the chef's bill. The numbers didn't lie—I was actually saving money by hiring a personal chef. I saved not only money but also time and energy, which I was then able to devote to my children and my writing! It cut down my grocery store trips from every day to twice a week. There were no more unused ingredients or food to throw out. I didn't have to spend money on spices, condiments, and ingredients that I might never finish. And the best part is that my son's weight remained stable.

How on earth can it cost less? Well, chefs typically cook for more than one family in any given city, so they divide up or share ingredients among different families. So instead of paying for a whole package of celery, I am only paying for the two stalks they used in preparing my family's meals. They also shop at farmers markets or buy certain ingredients in bulk, which can be considerably less expensive. All I have to do is pop the dinners in the oven to reheat them. PS: it's also much less expensive and healthier than eating out.

So while a personal chef may sound like an outrageous idea, do a Google search for your city and take a look at the numbers. Factor in that you will be saving gas money and time normally spent grocery shopping. It might just be life changing.

When to Consider a Meal-Kit Delivery Service

Meal-kit delivery services are popping up everywhere. Even Martha Stewart has one. These are companies that cater to a wide variety of diets and health conditions. They offer paleo, heart-healthy, diabetic, gluten-free, kid-friendly, vegetarian, low-carb, organic, and non-GMO meals and more. How it works is that you select the diet your family follows, tell them how many people you are feeding, select the entrees that appeal to you, and click. Next, a box (on ice) arrives at your door with individual cooking kits containing all of the ingredients you need for each meal, along with cooking instructions. Some of them even slice and dice the ingredients for you, so there is no shopping, no worrying about what to cook, etc. What is nice is that they send you the exact amount of ingredients you need for each meal, so there is no waste. This is a bit different than a personal chef, as you will be doing the cooking yourself, but it eliminates the need to figure out what to cook and to shop for ingredients, and it saves time because all of the ingredients are in one place with a recipe attached.

Again, I encourage you to do the math and give it a try. You may be surprised. Add up your weekly grocery bill, and compare the price of the dinner ingredients that you buy to what you'd pay for a week's worth of meal-kit delivery meals. Then try it for a week, and see whether or not your grocery bills go down.

If you decide to go this route, then I suggest ordering off either the paleo or low-carb menus; these would be closest to the meal plans I have created. You will just need to weigh the portion sizes to make sure they are appropriate. Most of them have nutritional information (grams of carb, calories, protein, etc.) available on their sites or included in the kits. *Today's Dietitian* recently reviewed several meal-kit delivery services, and of the companies that they reviewed, the ones I personally would try are HelloFresh, Terra's Kitchen, Chef'd, and Green Chef.

Again, working moms, single parents, parents busy with special needs, anyone looking to save time, or anyone who is overwhelmed by the thought of coming up with new ideas for dinner every night but doesn't mind cooking should definitely look into meal-delivery kits. You can order as few or as many meals per week as you like.

Decoding a Food Label

First of all, it's best to eat foods that do not have labels. That being said, there are four things that you should look for when reading food labels:

1. Grams of carbohydrate *per serving*. This should be 20 grams or fewer.
2. Serving size. This tells you what size portion contains that many grams of carbohydrate. Do not eat more than one serving.
3. Grams of sugar. You want to choose foods that have fewer than 5 grams per serving.
4. Do not eat any food that has any form of sugar listed in the first five ingredients.

Acceptable Sweeteners for Recipes

- Coconut sugar (limit 1 tbsp. per recipe)
- Raw honey (limit ⅛ tsp. for hot cereal or 1 tbsp. per recipe)
- Maple syrup (limit 1 tbsp. per recipe)
- Pureed dates (limit 1 tbsp. per recipe)
- Stevia leaf (limit to 1 packet per day maximum)

It is OK to use small amounts of sugar occasionally in cooking. More is allowed in a marinade if most of the marinade is thrown out and if it doesn't trigger cravings.

Avoid the Following Sweeteners

- Agave. Agave is not healthy. It is mostly concentrated, processed fructose (fruit sugar), which is turned to fat in your liver.

- High-fructose corn syrup. This is one of the worst things you can put in your child's body.

- Artificial sweeteners (aspartame, acesulfame K, saccharin, sucralose, neotame). Studies on animals have suggested a link between certain artificial sweeteners and increased insulin levels. People who consume artificial sweeteners are also at an increased risk of developing obesity and type 2 diabetes. In addition, frequent use of artificial sweeteners gets our taste buds used to things tasting intensely sweet, which makes natural foods seem bland in comparison. They increase food cravings, are *artificial*—man-made, created in a laboratory—and may cause a variety of health problems. Avoid artificial sweeteners!

- Sugar alcohols (xylitol, mannitol, sorbitol, and erythritol). These increase food cravings can cause diarrhea, gas, and bloating.

Shopping List

Nonstarchy Vegetables

Organic cucumbers	Avocado
Organic bell peppers	Jicama
Organic cherry or grape tomatoes	Organic broccoli / cauliflower / brussels sprouts
Organic carrots	Low-sugar tomato or marinara sauce
Organic vegetables/ salad for snacking	

Fruit

Organic blueberries/ raspberries/strawberries/ blackberries (in season)	Organic unsweetened applesauce
	Clementines
Organic apples/pears	Bananas

Meats and Cheeses

Sliced turkey (low sugar)	Chicken sausage
Sliced roast beef	Turkey bacon or pork bacon
Sliced ham	Chicken salad
Frozen turkey or pork breakfast sausage	Tuna salad
	Egg salad
Pasture-raised eggs	Fresh mozzarella cheese

Shopping List

Nuts/Seeds

Unsalted raw nuts (any type your child will eat)	Sunflower seeds
	Pumpkin seeds
Unsweetened natural nut butter (any kind your child likes; no trans or hydrogenated oils added)	Ground flaxseed
	Chia/hemp seeds

Hot Cereals

Unsweetened natural organic oatmeal or oat bran

Grains

Brown/black/red/wild rice	Mary's Gone Crackers or Flackers
Quinoa	
Wheat germ	Organic corn

Starchy Vegetables

Organic potatoes / sweet potatoes

Butternut/spaghetti/acorn squash

Frozen peas

Sweeteners

Raw honey	Stevia leaf

Shopping List	
Fats	
100% grass-fed ghee or butter Olive oil (dressing) Grapeseed oil (cooking at high temps)	Coconut oil or organic canola oil (cooking at medium temps) Shredded coconut Light or regular coconut milk (for recipes)
Yogurt	
Unsweetened whole milk yogurt (4% fat milk)	

Vitamins, Minerals, and Nutritional Supplements

Vitamins and Minerals	
You will need to supplement the following vitamins and minerals, as these food plans do not provide 100 percent RDA (Recommended Dietary Allowance) of all vitamins and minerals.	
Calcium Carbonate or Calcium Citrate	
4–8 years old	500 mg twice a day
9–18 years old	500 mg three times per day

Vitamins and Minerals
Vitamin D3 (Cholecalciferol)
600 IU per day minimum. Ask your pediatrician to check your child's vitamin D level and to recommend the appropriate amount of vitamin D supplementation. Vitamin D deficiency is quite common; most likely, your child will require more than 600 IU vitamin D per day. Levels should be rechecked after several months of supplementation to ensure your child is receiving the appropriate amount.
B-Complex or Multivitamin

Additional vitamins and minerals may be needed. Please consult with a registered dietitian or pediatrician for individualized vitamin and mineral recommendations.

Supplements That *May* Be Beneficial for Hypothalamic Obesity

The following supplements *may* be helpful in patients with hypothalamic obesity. Because there are currently no standardized recommendations on dosages for children and many of these have not been studied in children, it is very important that you consult with a functional and integrative medicine pediatrician, a pediatric registered dietitian, or a pediatrician who is knowledgeable about using these supplements in children and who can make proper dosage recommendations.

- Fish oil
- Alpha lipoic acid
- Chromium polynicotinate
- Magnesium glycinate
- L-carnitine
- N-acetylcysteine (NAC)
- Probiotics
- Prebiotics

Make sure any vitamin, mineral, or nutritional supplement that you give your child either has the USP, NSF, or Consumer Lab seal *or* is manufactured by a reputable, well-known company. This ensures that the products that you are giving your children are safe, high-quality products. Additionally, fish oil that is "IFOS-certified" means that it is free of contaminants such as mercury. I strongly suggest not purchasing vitamins, minerals, or nutritional supplements online. The manufacturers of these products cannot guarantee their authenticity, effectiveness, or safety when they are purchased from third-party sources online. There are many fraudulent and counterfeit products being sold this way; expiration dates are easily altered, and products are sometimes substituted with inactive or even possibly dangerous ingredients. Also avoid purchasing discounted supplements, as expiration dates are sometimes altered and sold at a discount. Always purchase nutritional supplements from trusted sources. Your health-care professional's office and small, reputable compounding pharmacies are among the best places to buy supplements.

Some high-quality vitamin, mineral, and nutritional supplement brands that we use in our home are:

- Kirkman
- Klaire Labs
- Metagenics
- Neurobiologix

- Nordic Naturals
- Ortho Molecular
- Pure Encapsulations

Eating Organic

What is all the fuss about? What does it even mean? A "USDA Organic" label means that food has been grown, handled, and processed without the use of artificial pesticides, artificial fertilizers, sewage sludge, artificial additives, hormones, antibiotics, or genetically modified ingredients. It also has not undergone irradiation or been chemically ripened.

Why is eating organic a good idea? Some studies have linked pesticides to cancer and neurological disorders. The EPA (Environmental Protection Agency) has established levels of pesticide residues that are considered "safe"; however, it is important to note that these levels are based on the studied effect that pesticides have on adults, not on children. Also, pesticide exposure will vary depending on how many fruits, vegetables, grains, and legumes you are eating. Children are much more vulnerable to pesticide exposure because they are usually smaller than adults, their brains and nervous systems are both still developing, and their bodies are less able to process and get rid of pesticides, especially if they have fatty liver disease.

Eating organic can be expensive. Fortunately, the EWG (Environmental Working Group) creates an annually updated list of the twelve most pesticide-laden fruits and vegetables, called the "Dirty Dozen," as well as the fifteen cleanest fruits and vegetables, the "Clean Fifteen." So if you want to buy organic but have to choose, you know where to put your money. It is also much less expensive to buy your organic produce at farmers markets and natural grocery stores. The fewer toxins that your child takes into their body, the better, especially if they have fatty liver disease.

Eat All the Colors of the Rainbow

Red, orange, yellow, green, blue, purple. The right kind of food is literally medicine. Try to get at least one food of each color into your child's body from fruits, vegetables, legumes, and whole grains *per day.* The more natural color you get into your body, the more phytochemicals and flavonoids you get, which are basically medicines from food that decrease inflammation, protect us from cancer and heart disease, and even improve brain function. Don't forget to limit fruit to two to three small servings per day. The following page offers some examples.

Exercise: Jump-Starting a Low Metabolism

The most effective ways to conquer a low metabolism are exercise that builds muscle, frequent small meals and snacks, and aggressive thyroid replacement (for those with hypothyroidism only).

Red		
Apples Bell peppers	Kidney beans Raspberries	Strawberries Tomatoes
Orange		
Bell peppers Butternut squash	Carrots Oranges	Sweet potatoes
Yellow		
Apples Bananas	Bell peppers Millet	Summer squash
Green		
Artichokes Asparagus Avocados Broccoli	Brussels sprouts Cucumbers Edamame	Green leafy vegetables Sugar snap peas Zucchini
Blue/Purple		
Blackberries Blueberries	Cabbage Eggplants	Olives Purple potatoes

Trying to lose weight without exercise is slow and frustrating; *exercise is a must*. While any form of exercise is beneficial and you should certainly do what you enjoy most (or dread the least), some forms of exercise are better at increasing metabolism all day long. Cardiovascular exercise, while important, increases metabolism while you are doing it, but your metabolism returns to baseline shortly after you finish. However, exercise that builds lean body mass (otherwise known as muscle) will increase your metabolism while you are doing it *and* cause your metabolism to remain higher for the rest of the day—even at night while you sleep! The more muscle mass one can build, the higher their metabolism will be. The reason for this is that maintaining muscle mass is work for the body, and whenever your body is working, it is burning calories. The body is constantly working to maintain muscle mass, repairing tears and replacing muscle cells that have died, so people with more muscle mass burn more calories while at rest. Fat tissue, in contrast, doesn't require any work on the body's part; therefore, zero calories are burnt to maintain it.

Let's take two people who are both five feet tall and weigh 120 pounds—Person A and Person B. However, Person A lifts weights every week and therefore has a good deal of muscle mass. Person B, who is the same height and weight as Person A, has very little muscle mass. Person A will have a higher metabolism than Person B; therefore, Person A will lose more inches and more fat and may even be able to eat more than Person B. Weight training, yoga, Pilates, barre, and resistance training all build muscle. It is still important to also get in some cardio, such as walking fast, swimming, running, bicycling, interval training, Zumba, etc. I strongly recommend hiring a personal trainer who can provide both the motivation and the supervision that young children need to exercise safely and effectively. This is the best place to put your money. Eating every three to five hours while you are awake also keeps metabolism high.

Most children with craniopharyngiomas develop secondary hypothyroidism due to the tumor invading their pituitary gland. The pituitary gland controls the thyroid gland, which controls our metabolism, so if the pituitary gland is damaged or has been removed, it cannot tell the thyroid what to do, which results in slow metabolism. It is imperative that physicians be aggressive with thyroid hormone replacement in patients with secondary hypothyroidism and hypothalamic obesity. Free T4 levels (thyroxine) should be kept in the top third of the normal range[1] in these patients to maximize their metabolism as much as possible. Symptoms of hypothyroidism should also be considered in titrating thyroid replacement dosage, not just numbers. There is also some literature suggesting that adding liothyronine (T3) *may* help increase patients' overall well-being and alertness.[2] Though this is not common practice, there are physicians who prescribe both T3 and T4 rather than T4 monotherapy in patients with hypothalamic obesity with secondary hypothyroidism. These patients report increased energy and increased ability to exercise.

The Value of Positive Reinforcement

There is a definite art to being controlling about your HO child's food intake but flexible when needed. For some people, avoiding all flour, sugar, and processed foods is imperative to keeping food cravings under control. For others, it is too restrictive and results in sneaking food, stealing money to buy food, or eating out of the trash. Let me give you an example.

A few days after we stopped eating man-made foods, I got a call from JR's teacher. She had found a bunch of food wrappers in his desk, and because she knew that I no longer sent him things like Goldfish and pretzels, she asked him where he got them. He admitted that he had

1.   Nathan C. Bingham, Susan R. Rose, and Thomas H. Inge, "Bariatric Surgery in Hypothalamic Obesity," *Frontiers in Endocrinology* 3, no. 23 (2012), https://www.ncbi.nlm.nih.gov/pmc/articles/PMC3355900/.

2.   J. K. Fernandes et al., "Triiodothyronine Supplementation for Hypothalamic Obesity," *Metabolism: Clinical and Experimental* 51, no. 11 (2002): 1381–3, http://www.metabolismjournal.com/article/S0026-0495(02)00099-9/pdf.

snuck back into the classroom during recess, pretending he needed to use the restroom, and taken another student's snack out of his backpack. Then, a few days later, another teacher found him finishing another student's lunch, which had been left unattended. The student was planning to finish eating once he was done playing soccer. After the second time in a week that JR stole man-made food, I realized that maybe the food plan was too restrictive for him, and therefore, I decided to offer him positive reinforcement for not stealing or eating other kids' food. I told him that each week he did not steal any food, he would be allowed to order hot lunch that Friday—whatever he wanted, even man-made food, as long as the portion sizes were reasonable. JR loved this idea, and he has not stolen any food since. He is so proud of himself when he gets to order his Friday hot lunch, and he looks forward to it every week. Sometimes he gets pizza or stir-fried chicken and vegetables with white rice. It is so motivating for him to know that he will be able to order hot lunch like his friends do, and it makes it easier for him to control his impulses knowing that he will get to eat something not on the food plan each week.

The other thing I decided to do was to send a big container of salad or cucumbers with avocado and bell peppers to school every day for him to graze on. His teacher agreed to allow him to eat it quietly during class. This was a clever way for me to hand over some control to him, but on my terms. Again, it worked beautifully and gave JR something to reach for when he was thinking about eating something that he shouldn't be eating.

So the moral is: if your child has HO, be hypervigilant and be controlling, but if you are so controlling that it is backfiring, then you need to figure out what you can do to give a little bit. Ceding a little bit of control goes a long way.

What to Do if Your Child Binges

What do we do if our child binges? It will happen. Should we then cut out food later in the day or the next day?

When you or your child slips, the best thing to do is move on, get right back on your food plan, and eat the next scheduled snack or meal. Skipping a meal or snack because of a binge will just lead to another binge or overeating later.

School Parties

Every HO parent's nightmare—the elementary school Halloween, Christmas/Hanukkah, and Valentine's Day class parties. It's like a sugar fest from hell. Donuts, cookies, cake, candy, juice, and fruit are almost always served. I find this so infuriating, not only because the schools and parents are overloading our children with sugar but mostly because it's such a stressful situation for parents and children with HO to be in.

Strategies I have used that have been helpful in these situations include the following:

1. I contact the teacher or principal about my child's situation in advance and gently inquire if they would be willing to set some modest guidelines. Schools are more likely to be receptive to practical guidelines, such as only one small serving of sugar-containing food per child, no juice, and no candy. Remind them that pediatric obesity is now an epidemic and that too much sugar can cause hyperactivity and behavior issues at school.

2. I sign up to bring the food for the class parties so that I can control what is served.

3. If that fails (as happens when other parents want to participate), then I find out in advance exactly what foods will be served at class parties.

4. I discuss with JR exactly what food will be served beforehand and ask him what and how much he thinks he should be allowed to eat.

5. If he insists on being allowed to eat more than I am comfortable
    with, then I counter that he may do so only if he skips his carb at
    morning snack that day and instead eats a double protein and/or
    does some extra exercise the day before the party. This teaches him
    what to do when he is older and wants to splurge.

6. I send plenty of nonstarchy vegetables with extra protein so that he
    has something else to eat to help distract him from taking additional
    sweets and carbs.

You can also just skip the party and take your child out to lunch or
to a special alone-time activity with you and give them a dark chocolate–covered strawberry or two. Explain that while it is OK to celebrate
holidays with a special treat, going to a party where there will be tons
of off-limits sugary food doesn't feel good (to the mom or to the child)
and that you love them too much to put them in a situation that doesn't
feel good.

Frequently Asked Questions

1. When it comes to nonstarchy veggies, we prefer raw, which I assume
    is preferred. What is the difference between raw vs. cooked vs.
    frozen?

Whether your vegetables are consumed cooked or raw doesn't
matter for our purposes; however, a combination of both is ideal.
The most important thing is that your child is eating nonstarchy
vegetables, so prepare them any way that your child is most likely
to eat or that you are most likely to actually get on the table. It also
doesn't matter if they are fresh, cooked, or frozen. While raw may
have a lower glycemic index, cooked nonstarchy vegetables are also
very low. Plus, cooking vegetables with fat, like oil or butter, helps
certain vitamins and phytochemicals to be more easily absorbed.

2. What do you think about juices, like freshly squeezed orange juice, pear, apple, etc.? Is this just like adding sugar/fruit to our diet?

    Don't allow your child to drink fruit juice. It is pure fructose sugar but without the fiber to slow absorption. Fruit juice is basically as unhealthy as soda for children with weight issues. You can, however, put whole fruits and vegetables into a blender and add 2–3 ounces of coconut milk or unsweetened almond milk. It makes a thick smoothie. This is OK, as long as you limit the serving size to 4 ounces, because you retain the fiber.

3. Am I correct in thinking that when I give my son a meal and he wants milk, I consider milk to be the carbohydrate and therefore don't give him any grains or starchy veggies with that meal?

    Yes, milk is considered a carbohydrate because it contains 12 grams of milk sugar (called lactose) per 8-ounce cup. I do not recommend allowing children with HO to drink cow's milk. Many people find milk triggers the same "reward center" in the brain as table sugar (sucrose); therefore, drinking milk is not a great idea for most children with hypothalamic obesity. If you do choose to give it to your child, then limit milk to one 4- to 8-ounce glass per day. In either case, you will need to supplement calcium and vitamin D.

4. I just found out by looking at my stevia box that the first ingredient is dextrose. Isn't dextrose a sugar? I don't even understand how the packets can have zero calories when they have dextrose. Should I stop using it?

    Good catch! Yes, you should stop using it. Most sweeteners add some sort of filler or additive to prevent caking and add bulk to those little packets. Usually, they use sugar (dextrose), sugar alcohols (erythritol), or, in some cases, silica. Real stevia leaf is green and contains no fillers. Again, one packet per day of stevia to sweeten oatmeal is the maximum amount that I recommend using to avoid getting accustomed to needing everything to be sweet. Once you get your child's palate used to less sweet-tasting foods, their cravings should decrease dramatically.

5. What is the difference between glycemic index and glycemic load? Should we be only eating low-glycemic foods?

Glycemic index refers to a number assigned to a carbohydrate based on how fast (or slow) that food causes an increase in blood sugar levels. Low-glycemic-index foods supposedly raise blood sugar slowly, which is good, and high-glycemic-index foods supposedly raise blood sugar quickly, which is undesirable. However, what glycemic index doesn't tell you is how high your blood sugar actually goes when you eat a certain carbohydrate, because it does not take into account how many grams of carbohydrate are eaten. Are you eating 4 ounces of a low-glycemic food or 10 ounces? It does make a difference. Glycemic load tells you both how fast your blood sugar will rise and how high your blood sugar will go. The higher the blood sugar, the more insulin is secreted to lower it.

But the truth is that using glycemic index/load is not quite that simple or reliable. Firstly, the glycemic index of any food stands only if you are eating the carbohydrate alone, without any other food. Once you add a source of fat, fiber, or protein or even cook the carbohydrate, the glycemic index changes anyway.

Recent research has shown that glycemic index may be an unreliable tool because there is quite a bit of variability in glycemic response in one person and possibly even more variability in glycemic index from one person to the next. That means that if I were to eat a piece of white bread (without any fat, protein, or fiber with it), my body could respond to it as a high-glycemic-index food at 10:00

a.m., but my glycemic response to the same food might be much lower at 3:00 p.m. Furthermore, if ten people eat a slice of white bread (again, alone, without protein, fat, or fiber), it may act as a high-glycemic-index food for some, a medium-glycemic-index food for some, and a low-glycemic-index food for others.

All of the arguments for and against limiting fruits, grains, and starchy vegetables to low-glycemic-index sources honestly make my head spin. Both sides make compelling arguments. The truth is that all of our bodies handle carbohydrates differently, not only overall but also depending on the time of day, our activity level that particular day, and changes that occur as we age. Some people are just more "carb-tolerant" than others.

Nutritional advice should be customized and should always meet the client where they are. Some people prefer to keep it simple and will just give up if too many foods are restricted. If you are one of those people, then don't worry about what the glycemic index of a fruit, starchy vegetable, or grain might be; just include all of them, weigh your food, and follow your food plan, which is a plan with a pretty low glycemic load as it is. Others want to use every possible tool to further their child's weight-loss goals and feel more comfortable serving only foods with the lowest glycemic index. That's fine too. Or you can try it both ways and see what works for you or your child. If, for two to four weeks, you disregard glycemic index or glycemic load (eat all fruits, grains, and starchy vegetables), measure all of your portion sizes, do not go off the plan, and exercise and still don't lose weight, then try one month of limiting fruit, whole grains, and starchy vegetables to low- and medium-glycemic-index sources. If you change nothing else (don't increase exercise or eat smaller portion sizes than before) and see weight loss, then it sounds like you may have found something that works for you. That's great! What works for one person's body may not work for another's, which is why it's impossible to give standardized nutritional advice to everyone.

That is all I have to say about glycemic index.

6. What is ketosis?

When we do not eat enough carbohydrates, protein, or calories, our bodies will begin to break down fat for energy. Ketones are a byproduct of this process of turning fat into energy. Too many ketones cause our blood to become acidic, and when that happens, we are "in ketosis." This is a nutritional ketosis, very different from ketoacidosis, which is a very dangerous condition that only people who have type 1 diabetes can develop. You can tell if you are in nutritional ketosis by checking your urine for ketones. In the United States, you can buy ketone strips over the counter in the diabetes supplies section of your local pharmacy.

7. What is a ketogenic diet?

A ketogenic diet is one that restricts carbohydrates to roughly 5–10 percent of total caloric intake per day, restricts protein to roughly 15–20 percent of total caloric intake, and relies mostly on dietary fat (roughly 70–75 percent of total caloric intake) for fuel.[3]

A ketogenic diet may make sense *for individuals with severe hypothalamic obesity who do not respond to a lower-carb or controlled-carb diet,* but only with the approval of your child's physician and only after you have tried to lose weight using a controlled-carb, no-processed-foods, no-sugar plan with exercise. Keep in mind that if one does lose weight on a ketogenic diet, then they will have to remain on a ketogenic diet indefinitely, even after weight loss is achieved, or they will gain it all back plus more.

---

3. "Ketones: From Toxic to Therapeutic to Ergogenic with Jeff S. Volek, PhD, RD," webinar from the Board of Certification of Nutrition Specialists' Second Annual Symposium, Nutrition Pro 2016: Personalizing Medical Nutrition Therapy, in San Diego, CA, November 12, 2016, https://nutritionspecialists.org/nutrition-pro-2016-videos.

I am not at all against trying a ketogenic diet for a child with severe hypothalamic obesity; however, it is not something that I can safely detail and recommend in a book. Again, true ketogenic diets cause a chronic loss of sodium, fluid, potassium, and other electrolytes that can be dangerous for individuals with diabetes insipidus, specifically those that do not have an intact thirst mechanism. Therefore, ketogenic diets should only be undertaken in those with DI under the direct supervision of an endocrinologist and registered dietitian who specialize in ketogenic diets and who understand the pathophysiology of diabetes insipidus.

To Lock or Not to Lock?

This is a tough one. At least, it was for me. The idea of locking the fridge and pantry was anathema to me. I couldn't even consider doing it. I knew that it was something that had to be done for many children who have HO with hyperphagia, but I simply could not accept that things had deteriorated to the point that we needed to lock access to food for a while. I worried that doing so would prevent my son from learning to control himself, that locking up the food would exacerbate his food obsession and lead to control issues that would make his food-seeking worse, and that it wouldn't be fair to his younger brother.

So I chose to watch him gain 140 pounds instead. Denial is a powerful thing.

Well, hindsight is twenty-twenty. Here is what I would advise the me of seven years ago. I would tell myself that children *with* HO *and hyperphagia* who are younger than ten or eleven years old are not developmentally able to control themselves around food. They are not able to connect eating to weight gain. They are not able to understand that gaining so much weight can be life threatening. They have no concept of how much weight they will actually gain just by eating the same foods that their friends and siblings eat or how being morbidly obese will affect their health and daily living. Young children with hyperphagia do not have the motivation to overcome the incredibly strong signals that their brains are sending them to eat, eat, eat. They are just listening to their bodies and avoiding discomfort. Once they are older, they are more likely to be motivated to overcome their hunger, to push themselves to exercise, and to take part in their own health and quality of life.

So my advice to those parents who have young children (with hyperphagia and HO only) is to lock it up and get over it. Rather than worry about how unfair it may be, remind yourself that you are helping your child and preventing horrible illnesses, constant fighting, and guilt. It actually might even be a relief to the child for you to take the temptation away, for them to be able to hand that over to Mom and Dad for a few hours at a time.

It is very important that you make your children a part of this decision. Tell them that the pantry and fridge will have to be locked to keep them safe and healthy. Not forever; just for now. Ask them what you can do to make it easier for them. When I asked JR this very question, he told me that he would feel better about it if I left some nonstarchy vegetables out on the counter for him to eat if he needed them. That was it. That's all he asked for. Locking the pantry and fridge when he was younger turned out to be life changing for us. It took away so much of the temptation, the anxiety, and the ugliness from our daily lives. There was no need to check his trash can for wrappers and crumbs. No need to have an anxiety attack several times a day when I found out that thousands of calories had been consumed on the sly. I was able to focus my attention on my younger child without having to keep an eye on the kitchen. I was able to take a nap. I no longer had to choose between hanging outside with the neighbors on a beautiful day and staying inside to watch the kitchen.

Once you have decided to lock up the kitchen, here are some vital tips to make sure that it actually works:

1. Install a Kwikset combination lock or similar onto your pantry. Do not use a lock with a key or the following things will happen:

    i.   Your child will find the key and binge on everything in the pantry while you are asleep or out of the room.

    ii. You will lose your key, be locked out of the pantry, and spend half of your day walking around your house, searching for your key.

3. Do not give young siblings the code to the combination lock. They will be put in a bad position when their sibling with hyperphagia begs them to open it for them.

4. Do not fool yourself into thinking that if you lock the pantry and fridge, you can keep a bunch of man-made foods in there, because there will be times that you or your spouse forgets to shut the door tightly or forgets to lock it altogether, and your weight-loss efforts will be derailed time and time again. *Keep the junk out of the house.*

Recipes

Here are some of JR's favorite recipes for breakfast, snacks, lunch, and dinner. Use organic fruits and vegetables and 100 percent grass-fed or pasture-raised meats whenever possible.

International Conversion Table	
Customary	**Metric**
1 cup	240 milliliters
1 ounce	28 grams
1 fluid ounce	30 milliliters
32 degrees Fahrenheit	0 degrees Celsius

Breakfast

Mini Egg Frittatas
with Yogurt Parfait

1 parfait = 10–12 g carb

Frittata Ingredients

- 4 pasture-raised organic eggs
- ¼ cup whole organic milk
- 1–2 oz. parmesan cheese
- 1 oz. sliced turkey, ham, bacon, or turkey bacon cut into small pieces
- Salt and pepper

Yogurt Parfait Ingredients

- 2–3 oz. plain, unsweetened whole-milk yogurt
- 2 oz. berries
- 1 tsp. hemp or pumpkin seeds
- ½ packet stevia (optional)

Frittata Directions

1. Preheat oven to 350 degrees Fahrenheit.
2. Grease mini muffin cups with oil.
3. Cook bacon or turkey bacon (if using).
4. Beat eggs, milk, salt, and pepper together.
5. Pour mixture into mini muffin cups, making each cup about half full.
6. Sprinkle meat and parmesan cheese, equally dividing them into each cup.
7. Bake for 20 minutes or until fully cooked.
8. Enjoy a few, and freeze the rest for another morning!

Yogurt Parfait Directions

1. Mix stevia (if using) into yogurt.
2. Layer yogurt, berries, and seeds into a 4 oz. cup.
3. Enjoy!

Breakfast

Fruit Smoothie
with Turkey Bacon
4 fl. oz. smoothie = 15–20 g carb

Ingredients

- 2–3 oz. unsweetened almond milk
- 4–5 oz. frozen fruit
- 1 tsp. ground flaxseed (optional)
- 1–2 oz. turkey bacon (uncured, no nitrates/ nitrites, no sugar added)

Directions

1. Allow frozen fruit to thaw for 5 minutes to soften.
2. Pour milk into blender first, and then add fruit and flaxseed.
3. Blend until smooth. If it gets stuck, add more liquid. Serve immediately, or freeze to make popsicles.
4. Cook turkey bacon on a skillet until crispy.
5. Enjoy!

Hot Oatmeal with Omelet
1 oz. dry, unsweetened oatmeal = 20 g carb

Ingredients

- 1 egg
- ½ oz. favorite cheese
- 1 tsp. grass-fed ghee or butter
- ½–1 oz. dry plain oatmeal (unsweetened)
- ⅛ tsp. or less raw honey
- ½–1 packet stevia
- Cinnamon
- Salt and pepper

Breakfast

Directions

1. Heat ghee or butter on a small skillet over medium heat.
2. Beat egg and pour into skillet.
3. When egg begins to set, add cheese and fold omelet in half.
4. Add salt and pepper.
5. Measure 1 oz. dry oatmeal into a small bowl.
6. Add boiling water (more for watery oatmeal, less for thicker oatmeal).
7. Mix in honey, stevia, and cinnamon.
8. Enjoy!

Grab-and-Go Breakfast   18–22 g carb

Ingredients

- ½ oz. pumpkin or sunflower seeds
- 1 oz. unsalted raw nuts
- 2–4 oz. fruit
- Chopped raw nonstarchy vegetable

Directions

1. Mix nuts and seeds.
2. Weigh fruit.
3. Cut vegetables.
4. Grab and go!

Snacks

Fresh Mozzarella
and Avocado Salad   15–20 g carb

Ingredients

- 10 grape or cherry tomatoes, sliced in half
- 1 bell pepper, chopped (optional)
- ½ avocado, chopped
- 1–2 oz. fresh mozzarella cheese balls, sliced
- 1 fresh basil leaf, cut into strips
- 1 tsp. olive oil
- 1 tsp. balsamic vinegar
- Salt and pepper to taste

Directions

1. Place ingredients in a bowl.
2. Drizzle olive oil and balsamic vinegar on top.
3. Add salt and pepper, and serve.

Snacks

Hot Dog, Fruit, and Cheese Kebabs
1 kebab = 2.5 g carb

Ingredients

- 1 uncured all-beef or turkey hot dog (without nitrates/nitrites), sliced into small circles
- 1 cheese stick, cut into cubes
- 3 oz. strawberries (or any fruit) cut into slices

Directions

1. Cook hot dog circles on a skillet.
2. String hot dog pieces, cheese, and fruit, alternating, onto 3 wooden kebab sticks.
3. Enjoy!

Cored Apple "Sandwiches"
4 oz. apple slices = 10–15 g carb

Ingredients

- 1 apple, cored and sliced so that the hole is in the center of the apple circles
- 1 tbsp. natural nut butter (without sugar or hydrogenated oils) or 1–2 oz. favorite cheese

Directions

1. Top apple slices with nut butter or cheese.
2. Put 2 slices together to make several small "sandwiches."
3. Enjoy!

Snacks

Watermelon Salad with Protein

4 oz. watermelon = 12–18 g carb

Ingredients

- 3 tbsp. lime juice
- 2 tbsp. olive oil
- ⅛ tsp. lime zest
- Fresh basil, chopped, to taste
- ¼ tsp. chia seeds or black sesame seeds
- Salt to taste
- 1–2 cups seedless watermelon, cut into cubes
- ½–1 oz. any protein

Directions

1. Whisk together lime, olive oil, salt, lime juice, and lime zest in a bowl.
2. Pour over watermelon.
3. Add chopped basil and chia seeds.
4. Cover and refrigerate.
5. Enjoy with protein.

Lunch and Dinner

Butternut Squash
Soup with Chicken Salad

6 fl. oz. soup = 15 g carb

Ingredients

- 4 lb. whole butternut squash (about 2 small squash or 1 large), washed and pierced
- 1 tbsp. canola oil
- 2 tbsp. 100% grass-fed ghee
- 1 small onion, diced
- 2 cups apples and/or pears (about 1 medium fruit), diced, peeled for a less grainy soup or with the peel to increase the fiber
- 1 small clove garlic, minced
- ¼ tsp. crushed red chili flakes
- 4 cups vegetable or chicken broth
- 1–1½ tsp. kosher salt, plus more to taste
- ¼ tsp. freshly ground black pepper, plus more to taste
- ½ cup either cream, coconut milk, or cashew milk
- ½ tsp. cinnamon
- ¼ tsp. nutmeg
- 1–2 oz. prepared chicken salad (store bought)

Directions

1. Preheat the oven to 400 degrees Fahrenheit, and place a rack in the middle. Line a baking sheet with parchment paper.
2. Coat the whole butternut squash in the canola oil and place on the lined baking sheet.
3. Roast butternut squash in the preheated oven for 1 to 1½ hours or until the squash is fork tender.
4. In a large, heavy-bottomed pot or dutch oven, melt the butter over medium heat. Add the chopped onion, and cook until the onions are translucent.
5. Add the diced apple or pear, and cook for 5 minutes or until softened.

Lunch and Dinner

6. Add the minced garlic and the crushed red chili flakes, and cook for 1 minute, until fragrant. Remove the pan from the heat and set aside.
7. When the squash is cool enough to handle, cut the cooled squash in half, and use a spoon to scoop the seeds out. Peel off and discard the skin, and add the flesh to the pot with the onion mixture.
8. Add the vegetable or chicken broth to the pot, and season with the kosher salt and pepper. Stir to combine.
9. Bring to a boil over medium-high heat, then reduce the heat to medium-low and simmer for 15 minutes, stirring occasionally to break up any large pieces of squash.
10. Remove the pot from the heat, and stir in the coconut or cashew milk. Let cool a bit until no longer steaming and add nutmeg and cinnamon.
11. Using a blender, immersion blender, or food processor, puree the soup until smooth. Taste and season with more salt and black pepper, if desired. Garnish with more cinnamon.

Hint: make soup for dinner, and use leftovers for snacks throughout the week.

Lunch and Dinner

Spaghetti Squash Fritters and Turkey Roll-Ups

around 4 small fritters = 15–20 g carb

Ingredients

- 1 spaghetti squash
- ¼ cup grapeseed or avocado oil
- ½ cup pistachios
- ¼ cup ground flaxseed
- 2 tbsp. wheat germ
- ½ cup grated parmesan cheese
- ½ tsp. kosher salt
- Paprika to taste
- 1–2 oz. sliced turkey (no sugar added)

Directions

1. Preheat oven to 400 degrees Fahrenheit.
2. Cut spaghetti squash in half lengthwise, and scoop out seeds.
3. Rub oil on skin, and place each half (cut side down) on a baking sheet.
4. Roast for 45–50 minutes. Remove from oven, and allow to cool.
5. Scrape out "spaghetti" with a fork. Use a nut bag to squeeze as much water as possible out of the spaghetti squash, and place squash in a large bowl.
6. Grind pistachios and grated parmesan cheese in a food processor, and add to bowl with spaghetti squash.
7. Add ground flaxseed, wheat germ, and salt to bowl, and use your hands to mix ingredients well and form small, flat patties. Sprinkle with paprika.
8. Heat oil in a cast-iron skillet and fry patties 3 minutes on each side or until browned.
9. Place patties on a baking pan, and bake for 5–10 minutes more.

Lunch and Dinner

10. Roll up turkey slices.
11. Enjoy!

Hint: freeze or refrigerate leftovers, and use throughout the week for snacks or meal carbs.

Chicken Parmesan with Sweet Potato "Noodles"

3 oz. sweet potato noodles = 15 g carb

This one is a family favorite!

Ingredients

- 4 skinless chicken breasts
- Tomato or marinara sauce of your choice (look for one that does not have more than 5 g sugar per serving)
- ⅓ cup ground almonds
- ⅓ cup wheat germ
- ⅓ cup grated parmesan cheese
- 1 egg, beaten
- Fresh mozzarella cheese, sliced
- 3 large yams, peeled
- 1 tbsp. canola oil or ghee
- 1 tsp. paprika
- ¼ tsp. salt
- Ground pepper to taste

Directions

1. Preheat oven to 400 degrees Fahrenheit.
2. Combine wheat germ, ground almonds, parmesan cheese, salt, pepper, and paprika in a bowl.

Lunch and Dinner

3. Pound chicken breasts until flat.
4. Season chicken with salt and pepper.
5. Dip each chicken breast into egg and then dredge in wheat germ mixture.
6. Place chicken on a wire pan grate (for extra crispness) or baking sheet, and top each piece with a spoonful of marinara sauce and fresh mozzarella cheese.
7. Place chicken in the oven, and bake for 20 minutes or until inside temp reaches 165 degrees Fahrenheit.
8. While the chicken is baking, peel sweet potatoes, and cut off each tip. Using a spiralizer or mandoline, spiralize sweet potatoes into thin "noodles" and set aside.
9. Heat oil in a pan, add noodles and 1 tbsp. water, and sauté until al dente. Keep stirring so that noodles do not stick to pan.
10. Place chicken on top of sweet potato noodles. Top with a spoonful of hot marinara sauce, and serve.

Lunch and Dinner

Grilled Ranch Chicken with Quinoa "Cakes"

2 quinoa cakes = 15 g carb

Grilled Ranch Chicken Ingredients

- ½ cup grapeseed oil
- ½ cup low-sugar ranch dressing
- 3 tbsp. worcestershire sauce
- 1 tsp. kosher salt
- 1 tsp. lemon juice
- 1 tsp. white vinegar
- 5 pasture-raised or organic skinless, boneless chicken breasts, cut into strips

Grilled Ranch Chicken Directions

1. Stir ingredients together in a large bowl, and add chicken strips.
2. Allow chicken to marinate at least 30 minutes (2–4 hours is better).
3. Heat grill to medium-high heat.
4. Oil grill with a high-heat cooking oil, such as grapeseed oil.
5. Place chicken strips on grill, and discard the marinade. Cook on each side until no longer pink inside or internal temp reaches 165 degrees.

Quinoa Cake Ingredients

- 1 cup quinoa
- 2 cups chicken or vegetable broth
- 1 large egg, beaten
- ½ tsp. salt
- ¼ tsp. pepper
- ½ tsp. parsley
- 1 tsp. oregano
- 2–3 scallions or 1–2 tbsp. onion, chopped
- ⅓ cup fresh parmesan cheese, grated
- ¼ cup flaxseed
- ¼ cup ground pistachio or wheat germ
- 1 large carrot
- 1 tbsp. avocado oil (not refined)
- Paprika

Lunch and Dinner

Quinoa Cake Directions

1. Rinse quinoa well.
2. Bring chicken or vegetable broth to a boil, and add rinsed quinoa. Turn stove down to low, cover, and simmer for 15 minutes. Allow quinoa to cool completely.
3. Combine the quinoa, eggs, salt, and pepper in a large bowl.
4. Place carrot, scallion, and garlic in a food processor (or finely chop) and add to bowl. Add cheese, flaxseed, and pistachio/wheat germ, and mix well. Allow mixture to sit for a few minutes in the refrigerator so that it holds together; add more flax and wheat germ if needed.
5. Use a ¼-cup measure to scoop quinoa mixture. Level flat, and dump out to form very small patties. Sprinkle paprika on top of each patty.
6. Heat oil on a cast-iron skillet over medium heat. Add patties, and flatten with spatula. Cook until bottom is crispy and brown.
7. Flip and cook until bottom is crispy and brown, checking to make sure they don't burn.

Lunch and Dinner

"Spaghetti"
and Meat Sauce   6 oz. spaghetti squash = 15 g carb

Ingredients

- 1 spaghetti squash
- 1–2 tbsp. non-GMO canola oil
- 1 yellow onion, diced
- 1 clove garlic, minced
- 1 lb. grass-fed ground bison or ground beef or ground pork
- 1 tomato, diced
- 1 jar marinara or tomato sauce (fewer than 5 g sugar per serving)
- Crushed black pepper and kosher salt to taste

Directions

1. Preheat oven to 400 degrees Fahrenheit.
2. Cut the squash in half lengthwise.
3. Scoop out the seeds, and place squash on a baking sheet flat side down.
4. Bake for 45–50 minutes.
5. Allow to cool enough to scrape the "spaghetti" out with a large fork.
6. Heat a large deep-dish pan over medium heat.
7. Heat oil, add onions, and sauté until translucent.
8. Add garlic, and sauté until fragrant.
9. Add ground beef or bison or pork, and brown.
10. Add tomato or marinara sauce, and stir until hot.
11. Add salt and pepper if needed.
12. Pour meat sauce onto 6 oz. "spaghetti," and enjoy!

Lunch and Dinner

Egg Frittata
with Potato Leek Soup   6 fl. oz. soup = 15 g carb

Frittata Ingredients

- 10 large pasture-raised or organic eggs
- 3–5 slices bacon or turkey bacon, sliced into small bits
- ⅓ cup parmesan cheese
- ⅓ cup whole milk
- ½ red onion, sliced
- 2 bunches spinach, leaves only
- 3 tsp. whole-grain mustard
- 1 tbsp. grass-fed ghee or butter
- Salt and pepper to taste

Frittata Directions

1. Preheat oven to 350 degrees Fahrenheit.
2. Whisk the eggs, mustard, cheese, salt, and pepper.
3. Heat ghee in a cast-iron skillet over medium heat, and cook onion and bacon until onion is translucent.
4. Add spinach leaves, and sauté.
5. Pour in egg mixture, and cook a minute or two until set around the edges.
6. Place skillet into oven, and bake for 20 minutes, checking with a fork to see if the center is done.

Soup Ingredients

- 3 large leeks (or a bag of frozen, chopped leeks from Trader Joe's)
- 2 tbsp. grass-fed ghee or oil
- 4 cups chicken or vegetable broth
- 2 lb. Yukon Gold potatoes, peeled
- ½ tsp. salt
- ¼ tsp. pepper

Lunch and Dinner

Soup Directions

1. Clean and cut leeks (or defrost). Cut off tough, dark-green tops, slice leeks lengthwise, and open each layer, running under cold water to rinse off any dirt inside.
2. Chop cleaned leeks.
3. Heat ghee in a heavy-bottomed pot, add leeks, and cook until soft.
4. Chop peeled potatoes into small pieces, and add them to pot. Add chicken or vegetable soup. Bring to a boil, and then simmer on medium-low heat until potatoes are soft.
5. Using a food processor or hand processor, puree into a smooth soup. Add salt and pepper to taste, and enjoy!

Nonstarchy Vegetable Snacks or Sides

Cheesy Roasted Cauliflower

Ingredients

- 1 head of organic cauliflower, sliced into large, thin slices (slice from top to bottom)
- 1–2 tbsp. avocado or grapeseed oil
- ¼ cup parmesan cheese
- ¼ cup gruyere or favorite cheese
- Salt and pepper to taste

Directions

1. Preheat oven to 425 degrees Fahrenheit.
2. Coat large cauliflower slices with oil, salt, and pepper, and place on greased baking sheet.
3. Cook for 30 minutes, flipping halfway through.
4. Add shredded cheese, and cook 10 minutes more.
5. Add salt and pepper.
6. Enjoy!

Nonstarchy Vegetable Snacks or Sides

Zucchini Fritters

Ingredients

- 2 large zucchini
- ½ tsp. kosher salt
- ¼ cup ground flaxseed
- ¼ cup grated parmesan cheese
- ¼ cup wheat germ
- ¼ cup finely ground pistachios
- 1–2 cloves garlic, minced
- 1 egg beaten
- 3 tbsp. avocado oil
- Pepper to taste

Directions

1. Spiralize and chop or grate zucchini.
2. Salt zucchini, stir, and let sit out for 10 minutes. Then use a nut bag or cheesecloth to squeeze out as much excess water as possible. Don't skip this step, or the cakes will be soggy instead of crispy!
3. Heat oil in cast-iron skillet over medium heat.
4. Mix the zucchini with the rest of the ingredients, and form very small and very flat patties. Don't make them too thick, or they will be raw inside.
5. Add patties to skillet, and cook on both sides until golden and crispy.

Nonstarchy Vegetable Snacks or Sides

Roasted Brussels Sprouts

Ingredients

- 1 bag brussels sprouts
- 2 tbsp. grapeseed or avocado oil
- 1 tbsp. balsamic vinegar
- ½ tsp. kosher salt
- ¼ tsp. pepper to taste

Directions

1. Heat oven to 450 degrees Fahrenheit.
2. Rinse brussels sprouts. Cut off tough end, and cut in half, then place in a bowl.
3. Add 1–2 tbsp. grapeseed oil or avocado oil, 1 tbsp. balsamic vinegar, ½ tsp. kosher salt, and pepper. Mix well.
4. Spread out Brussels sprouts on a metal pan, and cook for 20–35 minutes or until crispy but not burnt.

Nonstarchy Vegetable Snacks or Sides

Gazpacho
(cold vegetable soup)

Ingredients

- 28–32 oz. crushed tomatoes (preferably in a glass jar or non-BPA-lined can)
- 1 cucumber, roughly chopped
- 1 green bell pepper, roughly chopped
- 1 orange bell pepper, roughly chopped
- ½ yellow onion, chopped
- 1 clove garlic (optional), finely chopped
- 1 large beefsteak tomato or 4 plum tomatoes, diced
- 2 tbsp. lime juice
- ¼ cup red-wine vinegar
- 2 tbsp. extra-virgin olive oil
- 1 tsp. salt

Directions

1. Place crushed tomatoes, lime juice, salt, pepper, vinegar, and a third of the diced vegetables into a blender or food processor. Pulse until you have a coarse puree.
2. Place in a bowl. Add olive oil and the remainder of the chopped vegetables.
3. Taste, and add more salt, oil, and lime juice as desired.
4. Chill in the refrigerator for 2 hours (or until very cold) before serving.

Nonstarchy Vegetable Snacks or Sides

Summer Squash "Noodles" with Parmesan Cheese

Ingredients

- 1 large zucchini
- 1 yellow squash
- ½ tsp. paprika
- ¼ tsp. dried oregano
- Salt and pepper to taste
- 2 tbsp. grated parmesan cheese

Directions

1. Spiralize zucchini and squash.
2. Sprinkle with salt, and let sit out for 10 minutes in a colander.
3. Gently press noodles into colander to squeeze out excess water.
4. Cut noodles so that they are not so long.
5. Heat ½ tbsp. canola oil or 100% grass-fed ghee or butter, paprika, and oregano over medium-high heat in a skillet.
6. Add noodles to skillet, and stir for 1–3 minutes until soft but not soggy.
7. Move noodles to a plate, and add parmesan cheese.
8. Add salt and pepper to taste.
9. Enjoy!

Nonstarchy Vegetable Snacks or Sides

Jicama Stix

Ingredients

- 1 jicama, peeled and cut into sticks about ¼ inch thick
- Tajín spice to taste
- 1 lime wedge

Directions

1. Place jicama sticks on a plate.
2. Squeeze lime juice over jicama.
3. Sprinkle with Tajín.
4. Serve cold.

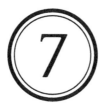

Chapter for Health-Care Professionals

This chapter is for registered dietitian nutritionists, physicians, and nurses, to aid them in treating and counseling patients with hypothalamic obesity.

Why Low-Fat Diets and Calorie Counting Do Not Work for Hypothalamic Obesity

In my experience, a low-fat diet, "MyPlate," and basic calorie counting are not only completely ineffective in this patient population but will most likely cause more weight gain and increased lipid levels. Hypothalamic obesity ("HO") responds only to a low- or controlled-carb diet that almost completely excludes "man-made" food (processed, sugar- and flour-containing food made in a factory). Why?

Fasting hyperinsulinemia is almost a given in patients with HO, and it is a large part of what drives the hyperphagia and weight gain to begin with. I believe that understanding this fact and knowing how to address it via diet was the key to unlocking my son's potential for significant weight loss. I stopped thinking of food in terms of calories or grams of fat and instead started to view all food in terms of its effect on insulin secretion. I also started looking at food in terms of whether or not it was "nature made" or "man made."

CDC Growth Charts: United States

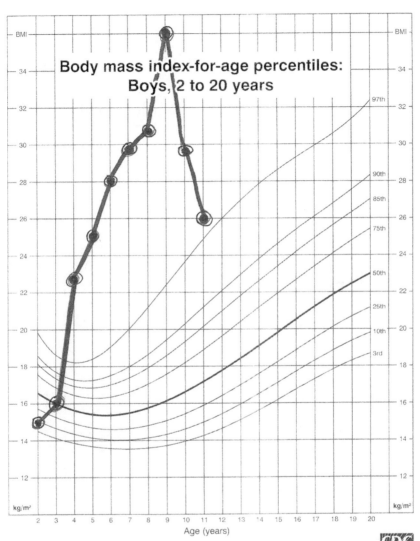

JR's change in BMI postsurgery.

Here is some information for you to think about:

1. Carbohydrates trigger insulin secretion. The more carbs one eats, the more insulin must be secreted to maintain euglycemia.

2. Continuously high insulin levels result in continuous hunger and fat storage.

3. Nature-made carbohydrates, which are inherently high in fiber, are more slowly digested and absorbed than refined or processed carbohydrates, resulting in reduced glycemic and insulin responses.[1]

4. High-fiber diets are associated with a reduced risk of diabetes and cardiovascular disease and improved insulin sensitivity.[2]

5. Protein does trigger some insulin secretion, but to a lesser degree than do carbohydrates.

6. Dietary fat slows gastric emptying, prolonging satiety.

7. Low-fat foods are higher in carbohydrate and therefore cause more insulin secretion than high-fat foods.

8. Low-fat, high-carbohydrate diets have been shown to raise triglyceride levels and to reduce high-density lipoprotein concentrations.[3]

---

1. L. Te Morenga, P. Docherty, S. Williams, and J. Mann, "The Effect of a Diet Moderately High in Protein and Fiber on Insulin Sensitivity Measured Using the Dynamic Insulin Sensitivity and Secretion Test (DISST)," *Nutrients* 9, no. 12 (2017): 1291, doi:10.3390/nu9121291.

2. Ibid.

3. A. Accurso et al., "Dietary Carbohydrate Restriction in Type 2 Diabetes Mellitus and Metabolic Syndrome: Time for a Critical Appraisal," *Nutrition & Metabolism* 5, no. 9 (2008), doi:10.1186/1743-7075-5-9.

9. Dietary fat has very little, if any, effect on insulin secretion.

10. There is a spectrum of carbohydrate tolerance. Some people are just more "carb tolerant" than others. Children with HO have a very low "carb tolerance."

So *why* on earth would we tell patients with high-fasting insulin levels to eat a low-fat diet? Low-fat diets are far too high in carbohydrate for a child with HO to handle. A low-fat diet guarantees more insulin secretion, higher triglyceride levels, and increased hyperphagia, which is what we are trying to avoid.

Looking at things from an insulin perspective, you can see how *not all calories are created equal.* Carbohydrate calories will cause weight gain much more efficiently in children with HO than fat calories due to carbohydrate's effect on insulin secretion.

Not only are calories not all created equal but carbohydrate calories are not all created equal. Nature-made carbohydrates cause less insulin secretion than do man-made carbohydrates because nature-made carbs contain fiber and/or fat and do not contain flour, sucrose, or high-fructose corn syrup. All of this lowers nature-made carbohydrate's glycemic index and therefore slows insulin response. In addition, because they do not contain flour, sugar, or high-fructose corn syrup, nature-made carbohydrate calories do not trigger food cravings, do not trigger over-eating, and are not addictive. Man-made carbohydrates do.

So *in the context of a low-sugar, low carbohydrate, high-fiber, low-flour, no-processed-food lifestyle, dietary fat should not be limited to any particular percent of caloric intake.* Liberalizing intake of dietary fat will promote weight loss, decrease cravings, increase satiety, and help patients stick to their food plan. Patients with hypothalamic obesity need to focus their efforts on limiting carbs and sugar, not fat. *Despite what you may have been taught, dietary fat does not cause weight gain and does not increase risk of heart disease; rather, processed food, sugar, and overconsumption of carbohydrates do.* Weight loss will decrease risk factors of cardiovascular disease, and weight loss can be more easily achieved by including fat in the diet and limiting the man-made and total carbohydrate. So forget everything you have been taught about dietary fat, weight gain, and heart disease. Dietary manipulation to minimize insulin secretion is the key to decreasing hunger and cravings and achieving weight loss in this patient population. The worst thing you can do is to recommend a low-fat diet for these patients. Instead, teach them how to carb count, to limit carbohydrates to 5–20 grams per meal or snack, and to avoid sugar and flour as much as possible. Also teach them the difference between real, nature-made food and man-made, processed junk.

More on Dietary Fats

Of course, monounsaturated and polyunsaturated fats and sources of omega-3 fatty acids—such as fish, avocados, walnuts, flaxseed, almonds, pistachios, nut butters, olive oil, etc.—should be encouraged over saturated fats. Trans fats should be completely avoided. However, saturated fat does not need to be so strictly limited. In fact, whole-milk *unsweetened* yogurt should be encouraged over nonfat yogurt, as long as the portion size is limited to 8 ounces or fewer. Drinking cow's milk and fruit juice should be discouraged, as they are high in sugar (lactose and fructose, respectively) without the fiber that slows absorption and tend to increase cravings in this patient population. Plus, cow's milk has the potential to be a huge source of excess insulin-stimulating calories in children with diabetes insipidus who like to drink cold milk when they are thirsty. Calcium and vitamin D should be supplemented. Fruit juice ends up being converted to triglycerides, contributing to elevated serum triglycerides and fatty liver.

To avoid behavior issues related to hunger, great things to snack on (between scheduled meals and snacks) are nonstarchy vegetables. Small amounts of dietary fat, such as 1–2 ounces of avocado, ½ ounce of nuts or seeds, olives, olive oil on a salad, or 100 percent grass-fed butter or ghee, may be added to nonstarchy vegetables a few times per day to enhance taste and prolong satiety.

What Kind of Diet *Does* Work for Hypothalamic Obesity?

1. A low- or controlled-carbohydrate diet that is made up primarily of nonstarchy vegetables, protein, and dietary fat; AND that limits nature-made carbohydrates to 5–20 grams per meal or snack; AND that almost completely excludes processed, man-made, sugar- and flour-containing foods (including bread, crackers, and pasta) is what works. This is because such a diet profoundly decreases sugar cravings and temptation and calms appetite in general, as well as minimizing insulin secretion. Please read section 4 of this book for a complete understanding of both the low-carb and the controlled-carb food plans for HO.

2. A ketogenic diet is a good option for patients with hypothalamic obesity *who do not respond to either of my food plans.* A ketogenic diet is not easy to follow. However, if a family is interested and motivated, I see no problem with them trying a ketogenic diet, as long as they understand that they will have to stay on that diet forever or their child will regain weight. (That goes for any diet.) Also, be aware that ketogenic diets cause natriuresis, which has the potential to cause sodium issues in patients with diabetes insipidus who do not have a thirst mechanism. Patients with DI should attempt a ketogenic diet only with the approval and supervision of their endocrinologist and, ideally, a pediatric registered dietitian who specializes in ketogenic diets. Sodium should not be restricted in patients following a ketogenic diet; in fact, an extra gram or two of sodium per day should be supplemented to avoid headaches, dizziness, and other symptoms of "keto flu," which is caused by ketone production. I have not included a ketogenic diet plan in this book.

Recommendations to Ensure Success

1. All high-temptation, processed, man-made, sugar- and flour-containing food should be removed from the home or kept under lock and key.

2. Limit fruit to two to three servings per day (4 ounces max per serving). This will decrease serum triglycerides and food cravings.

3. A maximum of three servings of 100 percent whole-grain bread may be permitted per week. This must be kept under lock and key.

4. Artificial and nonnutritive sweeteners should be discouraged, as they may increase insulin secretion and cravings. One packet of stevia leaf is allowed each day.

5. Children should not be allowed to drink anything other than water, unsweetened herbal tea, or the occasional nut milk or hemp milk.

6. A "special treat" of two to three *dark* chocolate Hershey's Kisses, five to ten *dark* chocolate chips, or similar can be given once or twice a week.

7. One small dessert per week of fewer than three hundred calories is allowed! This should be a high-fat dessert, such as a small donut, a single scoop of ice cream, a small piece of cake, or a small brownie or cookie (the size of the child's palm). If high-sugar desserts trigger bingeing or behavior problems, try a "paleo" dessert instead.

The charts on the following pages show how JR's triglyceride, cholesterol, and ALT levels have changed over time as his diet and lifestyle improved.

TRIGLYCERIDES - Past Results

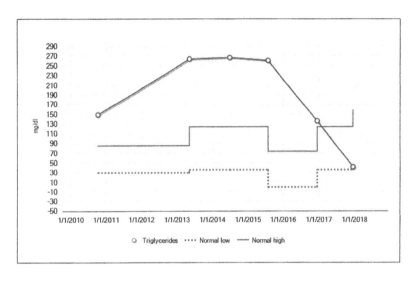

MyChart® licensed from Epic Systems Corporation, © 1999 - 2015.

Treating Pediatric Hypothalamic Obesity and Hyperphagia: A Seven-Pronged Approach

Diet is only one important piece to solving the HO puzzle. Failure to attack HO from several different angles will fail the HO patient.

1. Provide hope and encouragement to the patient and family.

    Choose your words carefully. If you tell your patients that HO is "unresponsive to diet and exercise," then most of them will give up before they have even tried. *It is imperative that you give them the gift of hope.* When one has a belief that something is possible, then they are more likely to summon the determination to make it happen. While patients with HO may always be overweight or even obese, with hard work and determination, it may be possible to "tame" their hyperphagia by following the prescribed dietary and

CHOLESTEROL LOW DENSITY LIPOPROTEIN - Past Results

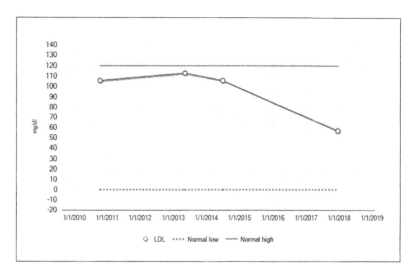

MyChart® licensed from Epic Systems Corporation, © 1999 - 2015.

exercise recommendations. *A positive attitude, some hope, a lot of encouragement, and clear nutritional guidance from the health-care practitioner can make the difference between these children being obese without comorbidities or being morbidly obese with nonalcoholic steatohepatitis, type 2 diabetes, and metabolic syndrome before they are eighteen years old.*

If you display a defeatist attitude to your patients' parents and give them the impression that there is nothing they can do, then you will kill any spark of drive, motivation, or desire they may have to encourage their child to exercise or try to control their food intake, because you are essentially telling them that there is no point in trying. I have spoken to countless HO patients' parents who have told me that their doctor told them that "there is really nothing you can do to stop the weight gain," so, therefore, they don't make their children exercise or try to change their eating habits, because what's

CHOLESTEROL HIGH DENSITY LIPOPROTEIN - Past Results

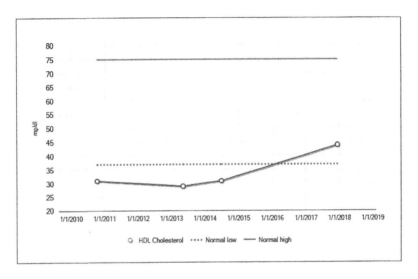

MyChart® licensed from Epic Systems Corporation, © 1999 - 2015.

the point? A little hope (and a lot of encouragement) might be all they need to motivate them to make some big changes that could make a difference in their health!

Of course, there will be patients with severe hypothalamic obesity that won't respond to diet and exercise—but we won't know who they are until they try! And in order for them to be motivated to really try, they must know that success is at least possible. Of course, older patients who continue to gain weight despite successfully implementing the diet and lifestyle changes that I detail in this book should be referred to a pediatric bariatric surgeon who specializes in hypothalamic obesity.

2. Instruct parents to set a weight-loss, weight-maintenance, or behavioral goal for their child, and offer positive reinforcement for meeting goals.

ALT - Past Results

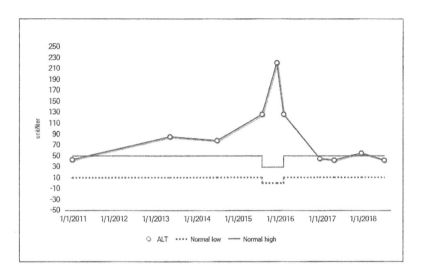

Positive reinforcement is very important in making this food plan successful, especially for children. If the child is not on board, this won't work. Parents must come up with a modest weight-loss goal, such as five to fifteen pounds or even simply weight maintenance, and allow the child to come up with some ideas for rewards that they can earn for sticking to the food and exercise plan and/ or losing or maintaining weight. Obviously, parents must agree to the reward or otherwise make some suggestions of their own. A visible line graph placed on the refrigerator, on which the parents track the child's weight-loss progress, is very motivating for all. Positive reinforcement in the form of high-sugar (but not fat-free) food or a meal "off the food plan" is acceptable and often extremely motivating for some children; for others, it can exacerbate cravings or food stealing. If this is the case, the parents need to switch to a nonfood reward. Nonfood rewards can be special alone time with parents, a vacation, extra screen time, or simply a toy the child really wants—whatever will be most motivating to the child.

3. The entire family must make the recommended dietary and lifestyle changes together. This must be a family effort, or the child will be resentful and resistant, and it won't work.

4. Parents should lock access to food twenty-four seven once the diagnosis of hypothalamic obesity with hyperphagia is made, especially for children younger than ten years old who are gaining weight rapidly.

5. Exercise is imperative.

    A combination of weight training and cardiovascular exercise is ideal; exercise should focus on increasing lean body mass in an effort to increase metabolism and insulin sensitivity. Weight training (under the supervision of a qualified personal trainer or parent), yoga, Pilates, and resistance training will all increase lean body mass.

    Swimming, weight training, water aerobics, gentle yoga, and chair yoga should be recommended to morbidly obese children who are new to exercise and/or have joint issues related to excess body weight.

    Personal trainers should be recommended if the family's resources allow. Personal trainers provide accountability, can tailor workouts to the individual's limitations and needs, and can prevent injury. Personal trainers can work with children starting at a very young age on elasticity, jumping, skipping, hand-eye coordination, medicine ball throws, and games that involve cardiovascular exercise. Children as young as eight years old can start learning and implementing proper form for weight training, although near-maximal training (heavy weights) is not recommended until postpuberty and into later teenage years. Even thirty minutes twice a week with a personal trainer can be very effective for these patients.

6. Maximize thyroid replacement for patients with hypothyroidism. If appropriate and safe, consider additional medication to maximize sluggish metabolism, decrease appetite, and increase energy levels.

Free T4 should be kept in the top third of normal range for HO patients with hypothyroidism.[4] Remember that basal energy expenditure in patients with HO is lower than in obese patients without HO, and *aggressive thyroid replacement is imperative.*

Consider adding liothyronine for HO patients with secondary hypothyroidism to boost metabolism and well-being. Some patients with HO who take liothyronine in addition to levothyroxine report that it increases their energy levels, enabling them to exercise. Remember that HO is an aggressive condition and needs to be treated aggressively; therefore, thinking "outside the box" is imperative to maximize quality of life for these patients. I am not suggesting putting patients into a state of hyperthyroidism. Just be as aggressive as you can safely be to counteract low basal energy expenditure and symptoms of hypothyroidism. While it may not be the standard of care to prescribe liothyronine in addition to levothyroxine, remember: these patients need all of the help they can get, as long as it won't hurt.

If you are not willing to prescribe liothyronine, stimulant medication may need to be considered to improve energy levels, which will make exercising more likely to happen. Once significant weight loss occurs, it is a good idea to discontinue stimulant medication for a trial period of a few weeks to see if it is still needed.

Be on the lookout for new research in the field of HO or Prader-Willi syndrome. One case report showed a reduction in weight and food-seeking behaviors in a child treated with *low-dose* intranasal

---

4. Nathan C. Bingham, Susan R. Rose, and Thomas H. Inge, "Bariatric Surgery in Hypothalamic Obesity," *Frontiers in Endocrinology* 3, no. 23 (2012), https://www.ncbi.nlm.nih.gov/pmc/articles/PMC3355900/.

oxytocin post craniopharyngioma resection.[5] Studies on oxytocin and multiple other drugs are currently underway.

7.   Controlled- or Low-Carb Food Plan.

Food Plan I is recommended for obese children and teens who have mild to moderate HO who are constantly complaining of hunger, who are stealing food (or money to buy food), and *who weigh at least 150 to 160 pounds.* This is the more liberal carb plan of the two. Nonstarchy vegetables may be consumed between meals without limit in this food plan. See Food Plan I in part 4 of this book.

Food Plan II is for younger children (minimum four years old) with HO, children and teens with HO who weigh fewer than 140 to 150 pounds, children and teens with HO who do not have hyperphagia, and obese children and teens with HO who do not see results (weight loss or cessation of weight gain) following Food Plan I. Very young children should use the lowest end of the serving size ranges given and increase as needed. Older or heavier children can use the higher end and decrease as needed. You may need to experiment with which serving size works best for your patients. See the food plan section of this book for Food Plan II.

Weight loss should not exceed two pounds per week after the first week or two, or their metabolism may be compromised. If they are losing weight too fast after the first few weeks, adjustments should be made by increasing protein or fat or by slightly increasing carbohydrates.

In order to produce and maintain weight loss, hypothalamic obesity must be attacked from several different angles!

5.   Eugenie Hsu et al., "Oxytocin and Naltrexone Successfully Treat Hypothalamic Obesity in a Boy Post-Craniopharyngioma Resection," *Journal of Clinical Endocrinology & Metabolism* 103, no. 2 (2018): 370–5, https://www.ncbi.nlm.nih.gov/pubmed/29220529.

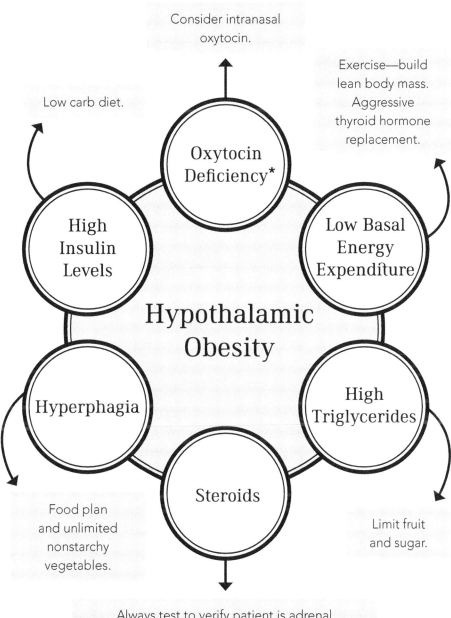

Consider intranasal oxytocin.

Exercise—build lean body mass. Aggressive thyroid hormone replacement.

Low carb diet.

Oxytocin Deficiency*

High Insulin Levels

Low Basal Energy Expenditure

Hypothalamic Obesity

Hyperphagia

High Triglycerides

Steroids

Food plan and unlimited nonstarchy vegetables.

Limit fruit and sugar.

Always test to verify patient is adrenal insufficient before putting them on cortisol replacement for life. Use lowest safe dose to prevent adrenal crisis.

* Research into oxytocin deficiency is cutting edge, and studies are ongoing.

Micronutrient and Supplement Recommendations

- Vitamin D in the form of cholecalciferol. Monitor levels before and after supplementation, and adjust as appropriate.
- Calcium carbonate or citrate, 500 milligrams two to three times a day. DEXA scans to monitor bone density in patients with adrenal insufficiency are recommended.
- B complex or multivitamin, containing 5-methyltetrahydrofolate and methylcobalamin.
- Fish oil, up to 2 grams per day, to decrease inflammation and triglycerides, unless contraindicated. Adjust dosage as appropriate for very young children.
- Monitor iron status and supplement if needed.
- Probiotic and prebiotic daily.

The following supplements *may* be helpful for children with HO, although there is currently no medical literature to support their use in children:

- Magnesium glycinate
- Alpha lipoic acid
- Chromium polynicotinate
- Coenzyme Q10
- L-carnitine
- N-acetylcysteine (NAC)

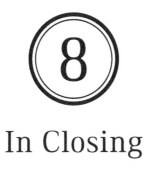

In Closing

Siblings of Children with Hypothalamic Obesity and Hyperphagia

One of the more difficult challenges that parents of children with hypothalamic obesity face in trying to control our very young children's food intake is this: they are too young to understand why their siblings are allowed to eat differently.

TJ (JR's younger brother) is an extremely picky eater; he has some sensory issues that prevent him from tolerating many textures. For years, literally the only foods he would eat were hamburgers, hot dogs, pretzels, tortilla chips, dry cereal, milk, sweetened yogurt, Goldfish crackers, and sweets. When I tried to get these foods out of the house several years ago, TJ was left with only about three foods that he would eat. It was an impossible situation.

Only one year old when his brother was diagnosed with this awful brain tumor, TJ has grown up listening to me and JR fighting about food all day long. He watched how anxious and upset I became each time JR ate too much or snuck food, and it had a very negative effect on him and his relationship with food. Food permeates every aspect of life, all day long—you can't escape it.

Not only was TJ forced to witness the constant fighting and crying over food, but the need to food police repeatedly pulled my attention away from him. It also took JR much longer to be independent due to the brain surgery. He needed much more help than TJ did with all of his activities of daily living. From TJ's perspective, everything was always about JR. The parties we could or could not attend because of the food that might be there, the restaurants we could or could not eat at, the trips we could or could not take—it all revolved around JR's hyperphagia. Plus, I was so tired and depressed for so many years that most of the energy I had went to caring for JR. I was racked with guilt over it but didn't know how to change it without compromising JR's health. I spent hours in TJ's room at night, reading and singing to him, trying to make it all up to him, knowing I was falling short.

I lived in survival mode for years. I lost my appetite as well and rarely felt hungry—only tired—and I often forgot to eat.

Not surprisingly, TJ began to develop food aversions. How could he not? His mother had no appetite, and his brother ate everything in sight, which made his mother upset. TJ gradually stopped eating foods he had previously enjoyed, and the number of foods he would accept diminished by the week until there were only fifteen foods he would accept, none of them healthy for JR. So, out of guilt at all of the time and attention I gave to JR and because I lacked the energy to fight about food with one more child, I ended up allowing these processed foods back into the house because I couldn't bear to see TJ not eat.

I tried to explain to JR that he couldn't eat the same foods that his brother could eat—that everyone eats differently and that what was OK for one person to eat could be dangerous for someone else. But JR was only five, six, seven years old, and he just didn't understand.

I had two children whom I loved more than anything whose needs were in direct opposition to one another. I couldn't win.

When I first started JR's new food plan for hypothalamic obesity, I knew it wouldn't work unless the whole family did it together. I knew from six years of experience that if I kept those high-temptation man-made foods in the house, JR wouldn't be able to resist them. So Dave bought a safe and kept some foods in there for TJ, and for a while, we allowed him to eat them when JR wasn't around. It broke my heart; I knew it was beyond dysfunctional and unfair. Yet TJ never complained. He "got" it. He learned quickly that if he mentioned the food he was allowed to eat to JR, it just made everything ugly, so he kept it to himself. What an unimaginable burden for a young child to carry!

As TJ got older, he began to get very angry at the kitchen being locked, at having to eat in secret, and at the general vortex of attention that his brother's needs created. I put TJ into feeding therapy and play therapy, which helped a lot. He slowly began to eat more healthy foods, which allowed us to decrease the dysfunctional "closet eating." Also, now that JR is older and his cravings are under control, he doesn't mind so much that TJ eats differently, and we are now able to keep a few minimally processed foods in the house (but only ones that don't tempt JR, like bran flakes and whole-wheat bread) so that TJ will have a few more things to eat.

JR's hyperphagia has been very hard on TJ. However, despite that, he has become the most extraordinary child. He helps his brother succeed every day by not bragging about the things he is allowed to eat when he is at school and by understanding that I cannot buy food that will tempt his brother. Now that TJ is older and JR no longer requires so much of my attention, I am much more comfortable telling TJ that he can choose to eat something healthy or he can choose not to eat.

JR knows now that his brother is occasionally allowed to eat foods that he will never be able to eat without compromising his health. It's still very hard for him, but he is old enough now to understand and accept that there will always be people around him—probably the majority—that will be able to eat things that he cannot. We have finally reached a place where things feel manageable with food again, where the focus is finally on TJ, and where we are all thriving in our own ways. Hyperphagia is tough on everyone on the family, but then, I guess, no family has it easy. We all just have different challenges to navigate. It's such a relief to finally have figured ours out.

Victim Mentality

So, you may be wondering, if I had the tools all along to control JR's weight, how and why did I allow him to gain so much weight in the first place?

The answer is complex and simple at the same time. I could go on and on about how exhausted I was, how strong willed JR can be, how I needed to have food in the house that my younger son would eat, how depressed and depleted I was, how hard it is for a health-care professional to objectively treat their own child, and how I worried that restricting JR's diet would cause an eating disorder. Those were all very real and very true. I had to work extremely hard to learn to replenish my energy by making self-care a priority before I was able to tap into my creativity and abilities. I first had to conquer the depletion, anxiety, and depression that had long prevented me from healing my child. However, I think that there was a larger theme at play: I had succumbed to a victim mentality.

What is victim mentality? It is an inability to move beyond self-pity and a tendency to cast outward blame for one's problems. I felt sorry for myself, my children, and the toxic family dynamic that the tumor had created. I accepted that since no one else knew how to help my son, I couldn't help him either. I blamed the tumor, the doctors, the pharmaceutical companies, even the pesticides and chemicals that I thought may have caused that tumor in the first place. This is what my victim mentality inner dialogue looked and sounded like:

The doctors aren't being aggressive enough; they're unwilling to prescribe medications that might help him! They have nothing to offer us, not even hope. There is food everywhere we go, and everyone else is eating whatever they want and enjoying themselves without consequences. Society has set us up to fail. The portion sizes are huge everywhere we go! Why force JR to exercise if hypothalamic obesity is not responsive to diet and exercise? There is no point in putting JR on a low-carb diet; it won't work long term because he will never be able to stick to it. He will never go along with it. He will never agree to eat vegetables or eggs instead of cereal and milk—why bother trying? His poor bother will have nothing to eat if I take away all man-made foods. My husband will never agree to eating differently. JR won't succeed because his dad will just keep bringing giant loaves of bread and pretzels and candy and pizza into the house, so what's the point?

I had a lot of excuses and a lot of defeatist self-talk when I was in victim mode. All of them added up and took the fight right out of me.

I spent six years looking outside of myself for a solution to JR's hyperphagia—researching and trying various medications to decrease his appetite or increase his metabolism, traveling out of state to see specialists, even counting down the days until he was a teenager so that I would be more comfortable with the idea of bariatric surgery. I looked to other dietitians and doctors for advice, and when that advice failed, I just accepted the idea that there was nothing left to try.

All along, I had the knowledge and tools to help him, but because I was stuck in the victim mentality, I couldn't summon the effort and determination to do everything in my power to help myself so that I could help him. So I remained depressed, anxious, and helpless, and I watched my son get fatter and sicker.

It wasn't until we were faced with the very real and imminent probability of JR not living to see the age of twenty that I was able to claw my way out of that victim "container," stop making excuses and blaming everyone else, and start to look inside myself for solutions, using my own intuition, knowledge, and education to help my child and teach him how to help himself. Once I did that, things improved so fast that my head spun!

Once I was able to shift to an empowered mentality and set an intention to do whatever it took to save JR's life, our entire trajectory changed.

Finding Contentment

Several years ago, my journey to find peace with my child's condition led me to enroll in a yoga-teacher training program. I had been not working for years, deciding instead to stay home and care for my children. I had lost myself in the process of caring for a sick child and in being a mother in general. I had been in love with and practicing yoga regularly for over a decade, so when my teacher decided to offer a two-hundred-hour yoga-teacher training program, I jumped at the chance to do something unrelated to nutrition that would give me both time away from JR's hyperphagia and something else to think about and focus on.

An important part of learning to teach yoga is to study and understand yoga philosophy. In Ashtanga yoga, there are two principles—known in Sanskrit as *santosha* and *aparigraha*—that really resonated with me. *Santosha* loosely translates to "contentment." *Aparigraha* means "not greedy or grasping," or, in other words, "letting go of your attachments." The idea behind these two concepts, as I understand them, is that it is our *attachment* to things (or people or ideas) that causes us unhappiness. Put another way, wanting what we don't have causes us to be miserable.

Wow. I mean, *wow*. I suddenly pictured myself miserably staring at family pictures that were taken before the diagnosis, yearning to have that life back, mourning the loss of the lives we had before the diagnosis. (It is very obvious which family pictures were taken before and after the HO hit.) I suspect that I'm not the first parent to harbor such thoughts after a devastating, life-changing diagnosis. However, the concept that it was my *attachment* to my idea of what our lives were "supposed" to look like that was perpetuating my misery was profoundly liberating. How might my life be different if I could only let go of my attachment to the life I had planned for my family and find contentment with the life that we did have?

These important concepts were life changing for me and allowed me to accept our new reality of medications, MRIs, tests, doctor visits, and hyperphagia. Could I be content with what I had? Was I going to continue to allow all of this wanting to make me miserable indefinitely? No. I was not.

I finally put those old pictures away in a closet so that I could focus on making the best out of "what is" rather than continuing to be depressed over "what was." They stayed in the closet for years. I recently hung them up again and am now able to look at them not with sadness and longing, but with pride. I once read an anonymous quote that said, "Your scars just show the world that you are stronger than whatever tried to hurt you." The change in JR's body portrayed in those pictures is just that to me now—a "scar" that shows the world that he is much stronger than what tried to hurt him. And that is what I think of when I look at those pictures now.

What I Learned

Having a child with a chronic medical condition is exhausting, stressful, and terrifying. It can also be transforming and full of hidden "gifts," depending on your perspective.

Some days are wonderful, full of smiles and small victories that are so much sweeter than anything a parent would feel at the success of a typical, healthy child. Some days are much more difficult. Some days, I am a stellar mom, patient and kind and focused on my children. Some days, I am so depleted or anxious that I lash out at everyone around me. Some days, I worry about the future. Some days, I grieve for what I have lost.

Having a child with hypothalamic obesity and hyperphagia has also led to tremendous personal growth. I know that I am a kinder, more patient and empathetic person than I used to be. I know what is important in life, and I have learned how to stop sweating the small stuff. I have learned that making sure that my needs are met is the only way that I can be the kind of mother that I want to be and that a tired, overstressed, overscheduled mother makes everyone miserable. I have learned some tremendous survival skills in caring for a child with such an all-consuming special need: I block out time every day to journal, to say aloud all of the things that I am grateful for, to exercise, to make sure that I remember to eat, and to take a nap without feeling guilty when I need one. I have learned how to say no to social obligations, parties, and volunteer work without feeling guilty. I have learned how to ask for what I need rather than expecting people to figure it out. I have learned to drastically cut down all the running around that is so depleting. I bring in support in the way of babysitters when I am having a rough time and need a break. I take a vacation when I need one. I allow myself to cry and to feel my feelings and acknowledge my fears. I have learned to let go of my wants and focus instead on how incredibly fortunate I am in so many ways. Most importantly, I have found my purpose in life: to use my degree and personal experience to help others with this wretched condition.

You Can Do This!

If you are reading this book and thinking, *There is no way we can follow this food plan; my family would never go for this*—I get it. I used to feel the same way. Other defeatist thoughts that contributed to my child gaining 140 pounds were: *I have another child, and it's not fair to him. I don't have time to cook like this. This will be too expensive. There is no way my husband is going to give up his chips, bread, and chocolate.*

Please don't wait until your child is sick, like I did. It is much easier to prevent weight gain than it is to lose weight. If this feels too hard or overwhelming, then I encourage you to remind yourself that this is what you have to do to save your child's life. This is not about aesthetics.

You do have the power to keep your child as healthy as they can possibly be under the circumstances. I am giving you the tools and the power to change your child's destiny. But if you write this off before even trying or tell yourself that the family lifestyle change that I am suggesting is too hard or that your child won't go for it, then please understand that you are making a choice—a choice for your child to perhaps become diabetic or weigh one hundred pounds more than they might otherwise. I don't care what your doctor told you or what you may have read in the medical literature about hypothalamic obesity, such as that "lifestyle intervention is essentially useless" or "lifestyle modifications are useless to prevent or treat it." That may be true for some, but not for all, and you will never know unless you try.

Please join my Facebook group, Craniopharyngioma Nutrition, which will give you a community of like-minded people who are fighting the same battle that you are and doing everything they can to win. I also post recipes, snack ideas, and relevant nutrition articles that will keep you motivated. Also check out my website, HungryForSolutions.com.

I fear that if I am not blunt, then I am doing you a disservice. If you think you have a choice in making dramatic lifestyle and dietary changes, make sure you understand what it is you are choosing. If you are worried that clearing out your home of all processed foods and sugar isn't fair or realistic or that it will somehow punish your family, then allow me to give you another perspective. You will be giving all of your children the tools they need to attain strong, healthy bodies and minds. You will be decreasing all of your children's risk of developing cancer, heart disease, obesity, fatty liver disease, and type 2 diabetes. You will be preventing them from becoming obese, sugar-addicted children and adults. You will be maximizing their brain function and energy levels. Clean eating is not a punishment; it's a gift. Real, nature-made food is medicine. Processed, high-sugar, man-made food is poison at worst and a recreational drug at best. True, it's not the kind of drug that will kill one immediately. It can, however, kill slowly, over decades. Should you really feel bad about keeping poison out of the house?

In Summary: Twenty Steps to Defeating Hypothalamic Obesity and Hyperphagia

1. Remove all high-temptation, man-made foods and foods that contain sugar from the home.

2. Remove anything that you or your child sneaks or binges on from the home.

3. Use salad plates for meals and dessert plates for snacks. This positively affects perception of portion sizes. Replace your bowls with

small bowls that hold no more than 10 ounces and your cups with cups that hold no more than 8 ounces.

4. **Exercise at least three to five times per week (preferably every day).** While all types of exercise are beneficial, weight training or interval training with a qualified professional will do the best job of increasing metabolism. This is one of the most important and effective things you can do for your child. It is money well spent and will save you more money in health care–related costs down the line. **Achieving weight loss without exercise is very difficult.**

5. **Make sure thyroid replacement is optional.** Free T4 should be kept in the upper third of the normal range to maximize metabolism.

6. **If your child has panhypopituitarism, make sure your child's cortisol and ACTH levels are tested** posttreatment and that cortisol replacement is actually necessary.

7. **Limit carbohydrate intake** to 10–20 grams at each meal and 5–20 grams at each snack, depending on the food plan you chose to follow. This will minimize insulin secretion, which will help your child lose weight.

8. **East mostly nature-made carbs.** Limit bread or bread crumbs to no more than three times per week, if at all.

9. **Do not allow your children to drink anything except water or unsweetened herbal tea.**

10. **Eat nonstarchy vegetables and small amounts of protein or fat between meals and snacks, if necessary.**

11. **Don't skip scheduled meals or snacks.** This leads to overeating later. Eat every three to five hours to avoid getting too hungry.

12. **Understand that sugar (sucrose, high-fructose corn syrup, and, for some, even fructose from fruit and lactose from cow's milk), processed food, and artificial and nonnutritive sweeteners increase food cravings and feelings of hunger and cause bingeing.** Do not eat any food that has more than 5 grams of sugar per serving or that has any type of sugar listed in the first five ingredients. One dessert per week is allowed as long as it doesn't cause your child to lose control. Desserts should be three hundred calories or fewer, so watch portion sizes.

13. **Do not eat "low fat."** Don't buy any products that claim to be low fat or fat-free, as they usually contain extra sugar and will impede weight-loss efforts. Remember, eating fat doesn't make you fat. Eating sugar and man-made foods does. *Especially avoid anything that contains high-fructose corn syrup or trans fats.*

14. **Don't eat out more than once per week.** Choose restaurants carefully. See recommendations for smart restaurant choices.

15. **Weigh all food on a food scale,** and do not go above recommended portion sizes. If your child is still hungry after eating, wait twenty minutes. If they still feel they need to eat, then let them eat non-starchy vegetables.

16. **Limit fruit to three servings per day or fewer.** This helps decrease cravings and triglyceride levels.

17. **Offer positive reinforcement** for meeting weight-loss goals. Set weight-loss goals that are not too intimidating. Five pounds, even weight maintenance, would be a good start.

18. **The entire family needs to avoid eating man-made food and sugar in the presence of the child with HO.** A child can't do this alone. Get spouses and siblings on board. Your child will be more successful if you are doing this together.

19. If your child has HO, their weight gain is rapid, and they are con-
    stantly sneaking food, **lock the fridge and pantry.**

20. **Exceptions can be made, of course;** everyone is different. Feel free
    to play around with what will work best for your child and your
    family. Small amounts of man-made foods may be eaten on special
    occasions, as long as this doesn't cause problems going back to the
    food plan.

A Dream Come True

So here we are, almost two years after this food plan changed our lives.
JR has lost forty pounds and has not regained any of it. His BMI has
gone from a morbidly obese value of 36.5 to a much healthier 25! His
health and quality of life have improved dramatically, and as long as he
maintains his current body weight as he grows, by this time next year,
his BMI will be in the normal range. His liver function tests are now
completely normal, indicating that he no longer has fatty liver disease.
He also no longer has high blood pressure, high cholesterol, or high
triglycerides. Although he *may* always be overweight, he is no longer in
danger of dying from fatty liver disease or any other medical condition
associated with obesity. His doctors are stunned and thrilled.

Most importantly, JR feels good about himself and what he has
accomplished! He is confident that he can accomplish anything in life
that he puts his mind to. He continues to exercise and was awarded
the Youth of the Year award at the renowned Cooper Fitness Center
in Dallas, Texas, in 2017 for making such dramatic health and lifestyle
improvements. The food policing that used to rule my life is now down
to a minimum, and we rarely fight about food! Our relationship is now
what a relationship between a mother and her child should be. *It's like a
dream come true!* We have even been successful at loosening the rules a
bit to allow him to eat the *occasional* breaded chicken, 3 ounces of pasta,
or even ten to twenty tortilla chips at a restaurant. Doing so has not
derailed his health, caused weight gain, or increased his cravings. We are

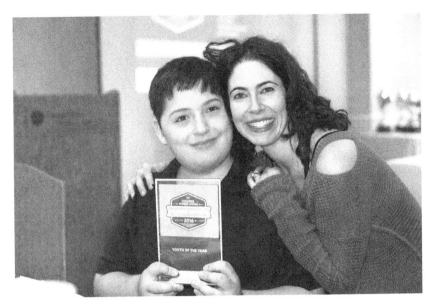

JR receiving the Cooper Fitness Center's Youth of the Year award.

now able to keep food in the pantry that we were unable to when he was younger, such as whole-wheat bread, nuts, and bran flakes, and he is no longer tempted by these foods.

JR has accomplished something that everyone, myself included, thought was impossible. Even with all the cards stacked against him— a slow metabolism, constant hunger signals, and high insulin levels—JR beat the odds through proper diet and exercise and the power of intention, hard work, determination, and family support.

If a child with hypothalamic obesity, a condition that is supposedly "unresponsive to diet and exercise," can lose forty pounds and keep it off for over two years, that means there is hope for your child too! This proves that not all cases of hypothalamic obesity are unresponsive to diet and exercise! Whether your child has hypothalamic obesity or is obese just from all of the man-made food that is poisoning our country, they *can* succeed in improving their health.

Acknowledgments

JR, thank you for being the inspiration for this book and for being so willing to share our story so that we may help others. I love you more than you can ever imagine.

TJ, your bright smile, your laughter, and your sweet, patient soul are what carried me through this. Thank you for understanding so much at such a young age and for being so supportive of your brother's efforts to beat this difficult condition. I love you more than you can ever imagine.

Dave, thank you for supporting my mission to bring our story out in the open so that we may help others overcome HO. You are my rock and my best friend. I love you.

Ray Ann, Mark, Shelly, and Steve, thank you for doing everything in your power to support us and, most of all, for putting up with me when I was the worst, most terrified version of myself. Dr. Michael Russo, thank you for being real with us. Your compassionate honesty was truly the catalyst for the lifestyle change that saved JR's life and improved our entire family's quality of life. Dr. Soumya Adhikari, thank you for being willing to think outside of the box to help JR be as healthy as he can possibly be, for all of the time you spend with me on the phone discussing JR's care, and for always making me feel like I am part of the team. You are truly a gift in our lives.

Dr. Siva Mohan, thank you for profoundly changing my life and helping me find my dharma. I could never have gotten through this without you. Ricky Tran, thank you for sharing the gifts of the Eight Limbs of Ashtanga Yoga, Patanjali's Yoga Sutras, and Yoga Chikitsa, which have helped me make sense of this life, given me great comfort in my darkest hours, and provided a healthy outlet for my body, mind, and spirit. Dr. Jeffrey Wisoff, thank you for your excellent continued care, your expertise and skill, your wonderful bedside manner, and for giving JR his best shot at a cure. Every day that continues to be tumor-free is a blessing, and we couldn't be more grateful. Dr. Tabitha Chansard, thank you for giving us the gift of hope; it has been life-changing. H. Theresa Wright, RD, thank you for mentoring me and teaching me about food addiction. This knowledge inspired my treatment of hypothalamic obesity and hyperphagia and enabled me to save my son's life. Shannon Edwards, thank you for teaching JR to enjoy exercise, for knowing just how far to push him, and for being such a strong role model and important part of his life.

Milli Brown, thank you for believing that my story should be shared with the world, for your support and guidance, and for making me feel like family. You are truly the neatest woman I have ever met. Tom Reale, thank you for your support and encouragement and for being so approachable, professional, and caring. Darla Bruno, thank you for helping me organize my thoughts and develop my story into something that I am proud of. Katlin Stewart and everyone else at Brown Books, thank you for keeping me on track, supporting me through a very difficult time, and helping me create this book!

Lisa Ronco, RD, CDE, CDN, MS, thank you for checking my math and for your feedback and support. Amy Wood, thank you for letting me bounce ideas off you and for your friendship and advice. Stacey Kaplan, thank you for your selfless support and guidance and your belief in my mission to get this book into the hands of those who need it most. Eugenie Hsu, PhD, thank you for keeping me company as we try to find solutions for our children.

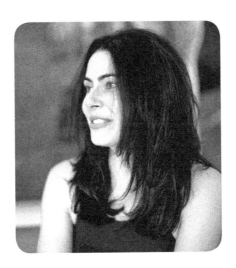

About the Author

Marci Serota earned a bachelor of science degree with honors in food science and human nutrition and an emphasis in dietetics from the University of Florida in Gainesville. She did her dietetic internship at Brigham and Women's Hospital in Boston, Massachusetts, and became a registered dietitian nutritionist in 1999. Marci worked as a clinical dietitian in the hospital setting for over six years and spent three years in private practice where she was fortunate enough to learn about and practice nutrition intervention for clients with food addiction, a condition with many similarities to hypothalamic obesity.

After taking some time off to care for her children, one of whom was diagnosed with a brain tumor at the age of three, Marci became a certified yoga teacher. Through her yoga training, Marci developed an interest in Ayurveda, the sister science of yoga, an ancient, holistic healing system that addresses the underlying causes of disease, the ways that we live, and what we put into our bodies. Through working with an amazingly gifted Ayurveda practitioner, Marci learned about using food as medicine. Marci has integrated this holistic perspective—along with her experience in treating food addiction and diabetes—into her nutritional approach to managing hypothalamic obesity. Marci's experience as both a registered dietitian nutritionist and as a parent to a child with hypothalamic obesity puts her in a unique position to help others who are dealing with this extremely difficult condition.

Marci lives in Texas with her husband and two children.